HELENA RUBINSTEIN'S BOOK OF THE SUN

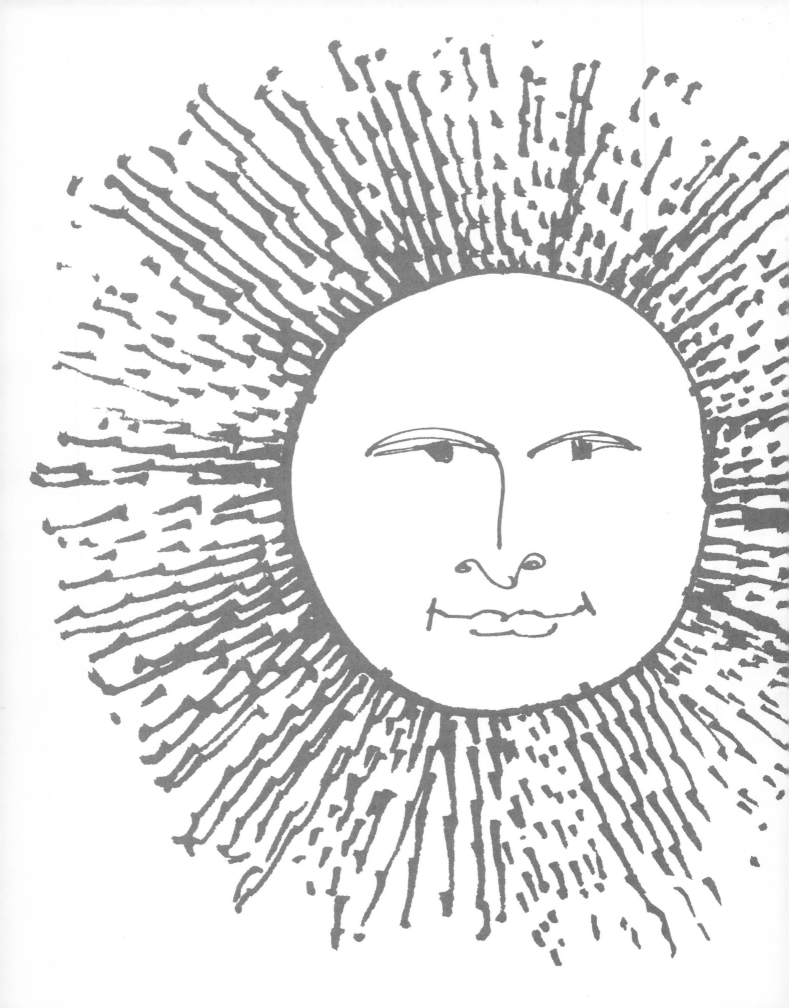

HELENA RUBINSTEIN'S
BOOK
OF
THE
SUN

Edited by Laura Torbet

Times BOOKS

Picture Editor: Barbara Rubensohn

Illustrators: *Paula Josephs*
Ronnie Kaufman
Kalia Lulow
Barbara Rubensohn
Laura Torbet

Editor: *Laura Torbet*

Associate Editor: Kalia Lulow

Series Editor: Barbara Bonn

Writers: Louise Weiss
John Foreman
Peter Skolnik
Sally Koslow
Kalia Lulow

Published by TIMES BOOKS, a division
of Quadrangle/The New York Times Book Co., Inc.
Three Park Avenue, New York, N. Y. 10016

Published simultaneously in Canada by
Fitzhenry & Whiteside, Ltd., Toronto

Copyright © 1979 by The Helena Rubinstein Company, Inc.

Library of Congress Cataloging in Publication Data
Main entry under title:

Helena Rubinstein's book of the sun.

   1. Suntan. 2. Skin—Care and hygiene. 3. Resorts.
4. Beauty, Personal. I. Torbet, Laura. II. Helena
Rubinstein, inc.
RL89.H44   613.1'93   78-20675
ISBN 0-8129-0809-0

Manufactured in the United States of America

Contents

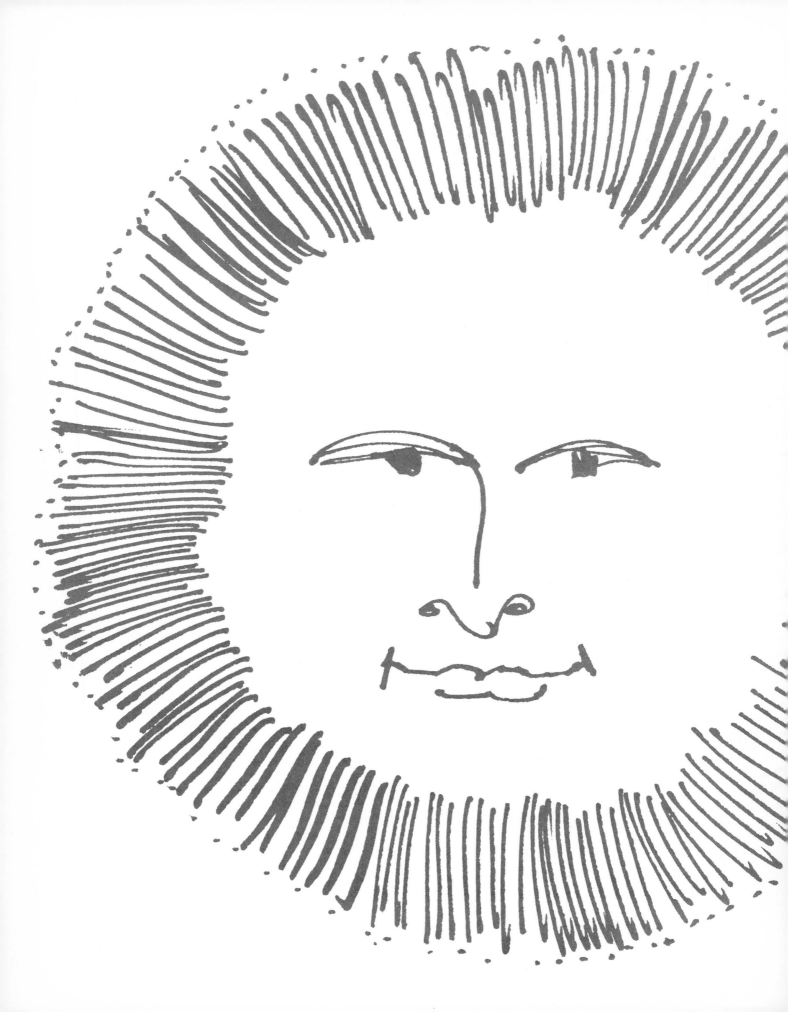

PART I
SUNNY HEALTH AND BEAUTY

I. All About Tanning

Shortly after the close of World War I, the legendary French designer Coco Chanel returned from a summer cruise on board the Duke of Westminster's private yacht. Always a trendsetter, La Chanel managed to transform this otherwise obscure footnote in the comings and goings of the leisured class into a watershed event in the history of fashion. You see, she came back with something that virtually no other lady of wealth or standing of the time possessed. She came back with . . . a tan!

In that vanished world tans were—and always had been—emphatically "out." Bronzed skin was not perceived as beautiful, primarily because it was prima facie evidence that its possessor had to work for a living. Not only work, but work outside, probably in a field somewhere. In the days before sports heroes, jogging, and cowboy fashions by Ralph Lauren, the outdoorsy image was *not* the one to aim for. It took free spirits with taste and, yes, daring to recognize the vigorous, beautiful look of tanned skin. Then these same people had to be rich enough to be able to lie down long enough to become tanned.

The fashionable rise of the suntan was one of the many revolutions in lifestyle that occurred during the turbulent 1920s. Titled Germans of the period, obsessed with physical fitness and the mystique of the ancient Greek Olympics, adopted suntanning with a vengeance. Soon tans and beautiful bodies became synonymous in the public mind. Obscure coastal villages on both sides of the Atlantic, as well as scores of forgotten fishing towns on the shores of the Mediterranean, began to see elegant summer villas rising discreetly on hills and along beaches. The people who built these summer places were quite visibly different from the generation that immediately preceded them. Unlike their own parents, they didn't wear collars to the throat or carry parasols on the lawn. Instead, they sported daring swimming costumes and possessed an equally daring determination to get brown.

So thoroughly has the suntan attached itself to the image of leisured and elegant living, that it remains to this day a highly sought-after and potent symbol of the good things in life. It is part of the athletic mystique in the summer and vibrates with the siren song of privilege in the winter. Privilege, that is, to exchange snow shovels, cranky furnaces, and runny noses for lolling around on some palm-fringed beach.

Everybody wants a tan now. At least it seems that way. It doesn't matter if getting one means baking on some sooty city rooftop or unaesthetic patch of crabgrass that you otherwise wouldn't dream of setting foot on. Because really, who will know just where you got the tan anyway? It's the color that counts. In fact, it counts so much to so many that we have spawned an entire generation (of women primarily) who have broiled themselves dark walnut every single summer for the last—well, maybe it's best not to even speculate on just how many summers they've been doing it. We all know these women. If we're really honest with ourselves, there are probably few of us who haven't

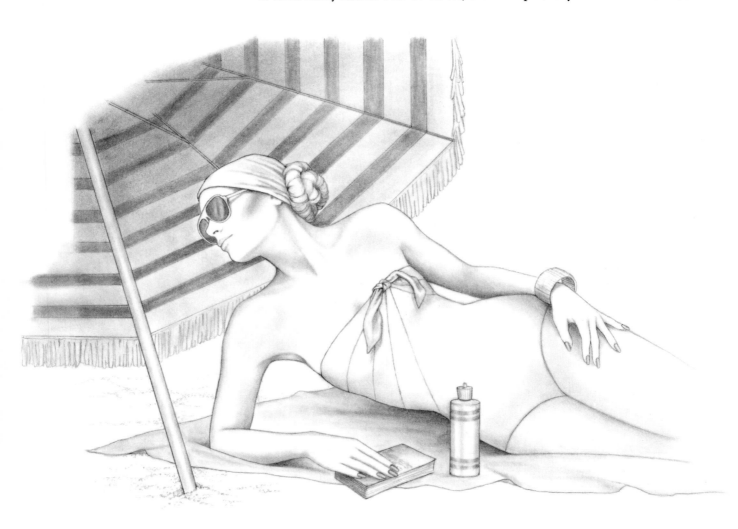

4

secretly envied them their gorgeous tans—especially when they turn up with one in February.

Regardless of the good looks of a good suntan, there turn out to be a host of dangers of which Coco Chanel never dreamed. Even though getting out in the sun is acknowledged to stimulate the body's production of vitamin D and the mind's achievement of a good mood, too much sunshine can be hell on unprotected skin. It leads to premature aging—slowly, to be sure, but surely nonetheless. That aging manifests itself as exaggerated sagging and drooping (called elastosis) and a prematurely leathery and wrinkled surface texture. There is also the constant threat of uncomfortable sunburn and unsightly peeling. And in extreme cases—no longer so uncommon—we have the threat of skin cancer, a disease wherein the growth patterns of sun-damaged skin cells run amok.

The good news, however, is that attractive tanning is perfectly possible without *any* of the above. In fact, thanks to today's cosmetic chemists, your chances of tanning safely and beautifully are better than ever. All it takes is a little education in the basic mechanics of getting a tan, a bit of caution on the beach, and a judicious choice of suntan products. To that end, we have devoted this book. And to begin with, let's have a look at suntans vs. sunburns.

SEPARATING TANS FROM BURNS

Tans and burns are decidedly *not* like the proverbial horse and carriage, love and marriage, man and his mate, or a good meal and wine. You do not have to get burned in order to get tanned. In Chapter 2, we go into specific detail concerning physiological changes that take place in, on, and under sun-exposed skin. For now, however, we'll just introduce some of the most important concepts relating to tanning.

The first of these concepts concerns the purpose of the body's ability to tan. Tanning is simply a defense mechanism. It enables the body to shield itself from potentially damaging solar rays. And it works quite well. People with good tans have a much greater resistance to painful sunburns than do those with alabaster skin. You've no doubt heard quite a lot about sunscreens. Well, your tan is simply your own natural sunscreen, which to a greater or lesser degree (depending on the tan) will inhibit the penetration of those damaging rays.

Suntans result from the release of the pigmenting substance melanin within the skin cells. This release is triggered by exposure only to certain of the sun's ultraviolet rays. Interestingly, the color of skin depends not on how much melanin it contains, but on how thoroughly that melanin is distributed within each cell. That's why black people, white people, and oriental people each have differently colored skin, but relatively the same amounts of melanin in each skin cell. The distribution of melanin—in other words, the color of your skin—is something you inherit from your parents. It can also be affected by sun exposure, which in effect stirs up the melanin in each new cell you produce.

A sunburn, on the other hand, is a phenomenon that really has nothing to do with sun-related melanin spread. Sunburn results from an entirely different group of ultraviolet light rays—about which much more information is contained in Chapter 2—that, in the absence of a protective tan or chemical sunscreen, have caused damage to the lower dermis layer of the skin. This damage includes the rupture of lysosomes, which are little self-destructing packets contained in human cells, plus the dilation of blood vessels and a resultant leakage of serum into the skin itself. This serum leakage causes blisters between the upper epidermis and the lower dermis layers of the skin. It doesn't matter whether you can actually see the blisters or not; they're still there. In cases of severe sunburn, the blistering is painful and apparent. But even where there's only simple redness and definite pain, there is still enough subclinical (i.e., unnoticeable) blistering to lead to the nemesis of all sunbathers—peeling.

Actually, your skin is peeling all the time. As plump new skin cells are formed by what's called the malpighian layer of the skin, old worn-out cells are simultaneously being sloughed off the skin's surface. This is a constant process of natural cellular turnover that keeps the skin renewed and supple. A sunburn, however, speeds your natural rate of shedding. The result is that the normal, unnoticeable sloughing of worn-out skin cells turns into unsightly shedding of sheets of undermined skin. None of this burning and swelling and peeling is inevitable if you: 1. get out of the sun before it has a chance to hurt you, and 2. protect your skin from dangerous ultraviolet rays by means of sunscreens and a properly developed tan.

STALKING THE PERFECT TAN: SIX VARIABLES

1. *Skin Type.* Everybody may have more or less the same amount of melanin, but the inherited distribution of that melanin within the individual cells critically affects your susceptibility to sunshine. The darker your skin, the more natural protection you have against sun damage. As you'll learn in Chapter 2, this damage is cumulative. It happens little by little, every time you go out in the sun. Much of it results from the breakdown of elastin, the substance that gives skin its elasticity (hence the name "elastosis" for droopy, sun-damaged skin). The darker your skin, the more efficiently you will be able to screen out exactly those ultraviolet rays that attack and destroy elastin. But even if you're black and particularly dark-skinned, your melanin will only partially protect you. No sunscreen, natural or chemical, is 100 percent effective against the aging rays of the sun. Fair-skinned people are even more susceptible to the damaging long-term effects of sunlight. For them, getting a tan is an endeavor to be conducted with the utmost caution, at least if future looks are a consideration.

2. *Time of year.* The intensity of sunshine varies considerably from month to month. It follows, therefore, that your chances of tanning and risks of burning vary correspondingly. In the Northern Hemisphere, the summer solstice on June 21 marks the highest and strongest point in the sun's seasonal transit of the sky. Sun rays—those that tan as well as those that burn—will be stronger on days that are close to the 21st, and weaker on days that aren't. It doesn't matter whether a certain sunbath falls on a day two months before the solstice, or two months after it; the intensity of the sun's rays will be the same. The point here is to realize that the sun's seasonal position in the sky is critically important for estimating the potential for tanning or burning.

3. *Geographical location.* The nearer you are to the equator, where the sun's rays enter at an acute angle, the more potent are those rays—particularly those in the ultraviolet range. Your chances of burning, or tanning, are twice as great in Fort Lauderdale as they are in Hyannisport, Massachusetts at the

same time of year. If you summer in northern Maine or Minnesota, you may have to work doubly hard to get your tan. Near the equator, by contrast, not only is the sun's angle more acute, but there is less ozone protection in the upper atmosphere. That means that the rays that reach you have less natural filtration. If you're planning a tropical vacation, you'll need extra amounts of sunscreening lotion, and you'll have to cut your normal exposure time often by as much as half. If the only people on the beach at noon are the tourists, it's too obvious a message to ignore.

4. *The reflection effect.* Black absorbs and white reflects. That's your rule of thumb when evaluating just how much sun you're really getting. This is because the amount of sunlight to which your skin is exposed is a function not only of the sun in the sky, but also of the rays that bounce off the ground. Thus, the more reflective the surface on which you tan, the more you'll need protection from the burning rays of the sun. Powdery white beaches are extremely reflective. In fact, if you retreat to the shade of a beach umbrella, you may still be receiving between 15 percent and 50 percent of the sun's burning rays by reflection, even though you're in the shade. By contrast, concrete only reflects about 5 percent of the sun's rays. Dry lawn grass is about the same as concrete. Gleaming winter ski slopes, however, are the most reflective of all. On a bright sunny day, a snowfield can literally double the intensity of the otherwise weak winter sun.

City dwellers are naturally protected—if you want to call it that—by air pollution, which actually screens out many dangerous ultraviolet rays. However, rooftop sunbathers, if the roof is high enough, will escape this filtering effect. That being the case, the rooftop itself or the deck or the towel on which you're lying must be evaluated accurately as to its reflective potential.

What about those hand-held silvery reflectors you see so often beneath the chins of sun worshippers? Well, if you value the future look of your skin, you're best advised to avoid them. The reflector may indeed give your face an early start on a summer tan, but it does so by concentrating ultraviolet light in areas that are rarely so exposed under ordinary circumstances, and therefore most likely to burn. Do you really think you'll be more appreciated for the deep color of your under-chin? Or the region under your nose? The skin on these fragile areas may even respond by tanning differently than the rest of your face. The result may be a tan that looks dirty around the edges. Besides, the reflected rays you pick up by just walking around in the sun take care of those areas perfectly well. The risks connected with a reflector hardly seem justified.

Water, incidentally, does not reflect radiation, but instead *transmits* it. This means, for example, that if you are swimming 3 feet below the surface of clear water, then ultraviolet rays are reaching you just as if you were floating on the top. Even at 60 feet beneath the surface, 1 percent of surface ultraviolet light will still penetrate. And the same applies to cloud cover. When the weather is overcast, time spent outside must still be counted as time in at least partial sun.

Ultraviolet light rays are determined to seek you out unless you stay inside or hide behind the car windshield. (Ultraviolet rays do not penetrate most window glass.) If you've exceeded the day's allotted exposure time but are determined to stay outdoors, then retire behind an umbrella, put on a sunblock (a description of which follows shortly), and sun glasses, and cover yourself in a tightly woven, long, loose robe. Don't gaze longingly at those cavorting in their bikinis. Think of yourself instead as mysterious and interesting. Besides, in the long run your tan will be better and last longer than theirs.

5. *Time of day.* Sixty-five percent of the sun's daily dose of ultraviolet radiation reaches the earth in the four hours around high noon. If your goal is a long-lasting tan obtained without burning, then you should initially limit your sunning to those hours before 10 A.M. and after 2 P.M. Once your tan is established, you'll better be able to withstand the noontime sun. The chart below will give you useful exposure guidelines keyed to your type of skin.

6. *Proper protection.* Never forget that the sun's effect on human skin is *cumulative.* Every single time its rays shine down on you—as you putter in the garden, window shop on the street, and sit on the beach—you are exposing yourself to ultraviolet rays. And certain of these rays will inevitably contribute to an aged appearance—*unless* you screen them out. Unfortunately, there is no product so effective, nor is there a tan so deep, as to provide complete, 100 percent ultraviolet protection. There are, however, plenty of excellent sunscreens that provide something on the order of 85 percent protection.

SUNSCREENS AND SUNBLOCKS

Before we describe these sunscreens and the ingredients that make them work, let's first differentiate between a sunscreen and a sunblock. The former has a selective effect, allowing certain tanning rays to penetrate freely while inhibiting others that burn. By contrast, a sunblock is an actual physical barrier that coats the skin with a substance impervious to all light. Zinc oxide is the prototypical sunblock; it's the white paste on the end of the lifeguard's nose. Cala-

GUIDELINE CHART FOR SUNTAN EXPOSURE

FACE:	First Day	Second Day	Third Day	Fourth Day	Fifth Day	Sixth Day	Seventh Day
Fair skin	15 mins	20 mins	25 mins	30 mins	unlimited	unlimited	unlimited
Medium skin	20 mins	25 mins	30 mins	35 mins	unlimited	unlimited	unlimited
Dark skin	25 mins	30 mins	35 mins	40 mins	unlimited	unlimited	unlimited
CHEST	not exposed	not exposed	not exposed	10 mins	30 mins	1 hour	unlimited
ARMS	15 mins	30 mins	45 mins	45 mins	unlimited	unlimited	unlimited
STOMACH	not exposed	not exposed	not exposed	30 mins	30 mins	1 hour	unlimited
BACK	15 mins	30 mins	45 mins	45 mins	unlimited	unlimited	unlimited
THIGHS	not exposed	not exposed	15 mins	not exposed	30 mins	30 mins	unlimited
LEGS	not exposed	15 mins	30 mins	30 mins	unlimited	unlimited	unlimited
FEET	15 mins	30 mins	45 mins	45 mins	unlimited	unlimited	unlimited

mine lotion and bentonite also work as sunblocks, as do long-sleeved shirts and pants.

Sunscreens are quite different from sunblocks. They don't look pasty and thick, and in most cases they will allow you to tan while still providing a measure of protection against burn-producing rays. Sunscreen products used to be based purely on a limited variety of partially effective chemicals. These included salicylates, anthranilates, cinnamates, phenyl, and benzophenones. With the exception of the benzophenones, these ingredients would allow the tanning rays to penetrate the skin while shielding (albeit imperfectly) the sunbather from many of the burning rays.

Then came PABA. This revolutionary chemical, whose name is an acronym for para-amino-benzoic-acid, is now contained in virtually every sunscreen, plus a good many sunblock makeups and formulas. PABA is far and away the most effective sunscreen ingredient that has ever been developed. It provides almost miraculous burn protection—so long as there is enough of it in the formula. To be effective, a PABA sunscreen must contain at least 5 percent of the chemical in a vehicle that is at least 50 percent alcohol. In fact, PABA requires an alcoholic base in order to stay soluble. Heavier bases require greater percentages of PABA in order to afford equal protection.

The great advantage of PABA is its amazing selectivity. Unlike benzophenones, for example, this chemical does not substantially interfere with those ultraviolet rays that lead to tanning. Instead, it screens out just the burning rays—and with wonderful accuracy.

Not everybody needs equal protection, of course. And this means, in effect, that not everybody needs the same amount of PABA. However, for long-term protection against cumulative sun damage to the skin, *everybody should be using some kind of PABA product.*

THE SUN PROTECTION FACTOR SYSTEM

How do you figure how much you yourself will need? Use the Sun Protection Factor system, which is widely used in Europe and has just been introduced in this country.

Developed by a Viennese professor, Franz Greiter, the Sun Protection Factor (SPF) is a numerical code assigned to specific sun products. This code enables you to determine almost exactly how long those products will be able to protect you from sunburn. We refer you to the SPF chart that appears on page 10. From it you can see just how long various skin types can be exposed to the sun without protection, and then how much the exposure time can be extended by use of products with various SPFs. For example, if you are a fair-skinned blond who, according to the chart, would begin to burn after 15 minutes of unprotected exposure time, then a sun product with an SPF rating of 2 would enable you to stay in the sun without burning for 30 minutes, or twice as long as you could without the product. Likewise, a product rated 4 would allow you to stay out four times as long, a hour in the case of a pale blond, but longer for other complexion types. A product rated 6 would give you six times the exposure, and so on to a maximum of 15. Anything higher than 12, however, is virtually a sunblock.

An advisory panel of the U.S. Food and Drug Administration, engaged in

SUN PROTECTION FACTOR CHART

SKIN TYPE		
Very Fair	Nearly always burns	
Medium	Often burns before tanning	
Dark (olive)	Skin that tans easily, rarely burns	

SUN EXPOSURE			
Skin type	Fair	Medium	Dark
You would start to burn within	15 minutes	20 minutes	25 minutes

USING FACTORED PRODUCTS YOU CAN STAY IN THE SUN			
Factor 2	30 minutes	40 minutes	50 minutes
Factor 4	1 hour	1 hour 20 minutes	1 hour 40 minutes
Factor 6	1½ hours	2 hours	2½ hours
Factor 8	2 hours	2 hours 40 minutes	3 hours 20 minutes
Factor 10	2½ hours	3 hours 20 minutes	4 hours 10 minutes

NOTE: 1. Start tanning gradually, avoiding the hours between 10 A.M. and 2 P.M. Add no more than 5 minutes daily to your tanning schedule.
2. Always use a higher factored product on easily burned areas, such as nose, lower lip, ears, etc.
3. Follow directions carefully. Apply sunscreens before going into the sun.
4. When you want a light tan, use a high factored product.
5. Reapply any sunscreen after swimming, exercise, perspiring.

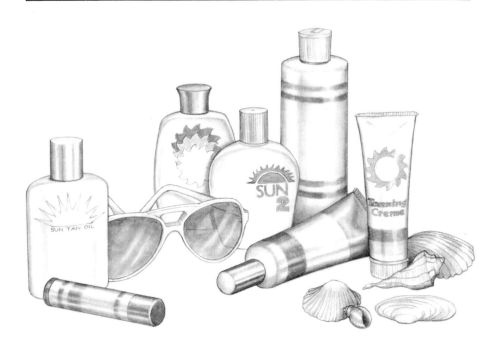

a study of drugs sold over the counter, has recommended that all sun tanning products be evaluated in terms of Sun Protection Factor (SPF) and display these numbers prominently on the tube or bottle. But at the moment, although some companies have already adopted the system, the purchaser must still play detective. One clue in trying to determine just how much protection you're getting is the product title. Words like "screening" or "blocking" are usually included when there is a serious effort to put a veil between you and a sunburn. However, "tanning cream," "sun lotion," and similar vague labels often mean you are dealing with nothing more than a skin soother. It may feel pleasant on the skin, but it will do nothing to prevent sunburning in any way. The only way you can be sure is to scan the ingredients list for the chemical names mentioned earlier.

In deciding the Sun Protection Factor number best suited to your type of skin, bear in mind your past sunning history. Does a half-hour exposure to an early June sun in mid-afternoon turn you beet red? Maybe its your Celtic blood. You should select a product with a high protection factor and follow directions to the letter. It may take you a while to tan, but a slow tan is better than a fast burn. So you should at least start the season with a product bearing an SPF of, say, 8. On the other hand, maybe you're always the first on your block with the deepest tan without any conscious effort at all. In that case you can start the summer tanning season with a lower SPF, perhaps one with a 4.

Once you establish your base tan, then you may want to change over to a product with a lower SPF. There's nothing wrong with this, since your own carefully developed tan will make up for the lower level of product protection. In some cases, however, you are well advised to stick with a high SPF sunscreen throughout the summer, regardless of the progress of your tan. Cases like this include people who have photosensitive reactions when exposed to sunlight (triggered usually by systemic medications, many of which are discussed in Chapter 2); or women who tend to develop chloasma, the darkening of facial pigmentation caused by sunlight in combination either with birth-control pills or with pregnancy.

Our final warning on the subject of proper protection is not to hurry. Patience always pays off in terms of long-lasting tanning. Remember, tanned skin results from melanin distribution in newly formed cells that must work their way up to the skin's surface. Your top layer of skin cells is already flaking off. Tans don't really fade, they flake away. And needless sunburns only hurry the flaking process.

NEW DEVELOPMENTS IN TANNING SCIENCE

PABA and the Sun Protection Factor system have made tanning surer and safer for us all. But until recently a couple of the most stubborn suntanning questions remained unanswered:

Is there any way to safely speed up the tanning process without increased danger of burning, and to more quickly put a tan barrier between our bodies and the burning rays of the sun?

Is there any way to enhance our genetic ability to tan and to get a darker tan than usual?

Well, it seems that as this book goes to press, the answer to both questions is yes. Yes, because a new tanning discovery attacks the problems at the source—the production and distribution of our bodies' melanin. The latest suntan formulations contain a rather remarkable new substance that induces and accelerates increased melanin production by the body in response to the sun's rays. The result is that you tan not only faster, but also darker. Of course, the new melanin-accelerating products contain the usual PABA and other sunscreens and are rated according to the Sun Protection Factor system. So you get the same protection against unwanted burn, with the added benefit of a more quickly acquired tan to put between you and the burning rays. The real bonus is a deeper, more beautiful tan than you believed was possible for your skin!

A FEW WORDS ABOUT PACKAGING

Suntanning preparations come in a variety of forms—lotions, gels, creams, oils, and foams—and an equal variety of packages—tubes, jars, bottles, aerosols, etc. The aerosols are probably the least practical for warm weather use, since special care is required to assure that they never reach a temperature greater than 120 degrees Fahrenheit, at which point they might explode. In addition, the effect of certain aerosol propellants on the ozone layer remains uncertain. So, unless their convenience strikes you as an overwhelming consideration, it's wisest to select another form of packaging.

The only other questionable packaging concept is the removable top on a

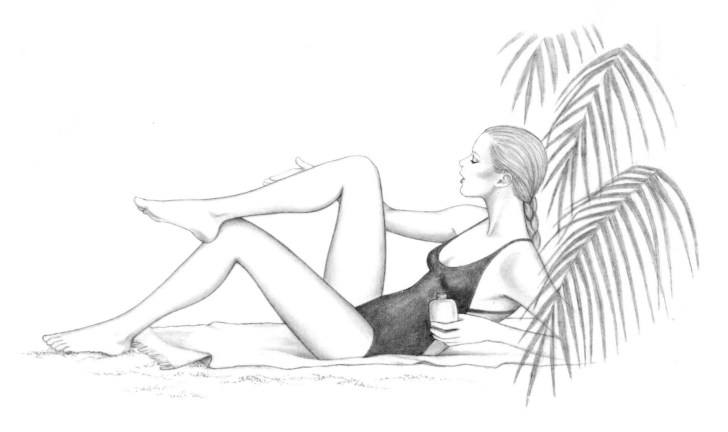

plastic container, which can easily fall in sand or snow. These two caveats aside, packaging is a matter of personal convenience, as are the vehicles, which vary from oil to gel to cream to lotion. Oils, gels, and butters feel greasy and tend to pick up sand particles. On the other hand, they stick well and make the skin gleam. Creams and lotions feel much the same as a light moisturizer, and you'll be less aware of their presence on the body. Clear liquids have a slightly oily feel on first application, but dry quickly and become unnoticeable.

SOME THOUGHTS ON APPLICATION

The oilier the preparation, the longer it's likely to stay on your skin. PABA adheres very well. But every sun product must be reapplied continuously, since they all tend to wash away when exposed to water or inevitable perspiration.

Surprisingly, there's quite a variety of application instructions on sun product labels. Some tell you to put them on as much as an hour prior to sun exposure to allow time for absorption into the skin. Others must be reapplied every two hours or after every swim. If you plan strenuous activity, such as tennis or volleyball, a product containing PABA is the winner since it's less likely to be washed off by honest sweat.

Leave yourself enough time for careful, leisurely application. The more even your tan, the less chance of peeling. This isn't as easy as it sounds because some of your body will be receiving more of the sun's direct rays than other parts, unless you have the patience to lie absolutely flat, turning every so often like a piece of meat on a spit. Actually, that kind of sunning has its own hazards. Those parts of you that are rarely exposed to the sun are most susceptible to burning. If you are going to be sitting upright or walking a lot, apply your sunscreen more thickly (or use a sunblock) where you'll be getting the brunt of the sun. These areas include the nose, lower lip, tops of ears, top of shoulders, chest, knees, and tops of the feet.

SUNNING IN (OR NEARLY IN) THE BUFF

We live in an era of body awareness, and the notion of nude sunbathing has recently gained a great appeal. Those who've tried both skinny dipping and nude sunbathing say the two have much in common, specifically, a delicious sensation of freedom.

If you can arrange a private, secluded spot, such as a terrace, backyard, or friend's poolside, you can get a headstart on your tan before deciding whether to brave it on a nude beach. Since you'll be dealing with skin that has probably been protected by clothing ever since you left diapers, all the admonitions about avoiding the noonday sun and using a sunscreen with a high protection factor apply doubly. It's one thing to show up at work or at the supermarket with peeling shoulders, but quite another to be unable to sit down due to burnt buttocks. Keep in mind the June 21 date as the most potentially dangerous, and begin at least a month before or after, when exposing the heretofore unexposed.

If you'll be sitting up, the tops of breasts or genitals will be getting the brunt of the ultraviolet rays. Apply the heaviest coating of sunscreen here, or perhaps a different, higher-factored sun preparation. If you'll be walking around, the buttocks will be similarly vulnerable. The area around the nipple, called the areola, has more pigment than the rest of the bosom, as does the nipple, so it will rarely need any special attention.

Women who expose their breasts to the sun often wonder if there's a connection between breast cancer and nude sunbathing. Well, don't worry. There isn't.

Should you decide to look into nude sunbathing in earnest, the options are many. Most nudist organizations are a far cry from a swinging singles image. They tend instead to be dedicated to lofty ideals, like world understanding and wholesome family life.

SUNLAMP TANNING

Sunlamps are a mixed blessing. It is indeed possible to maintain a tan or keep a rosy glow all winter, if you are careful. It is also possible to give yourself so severe a burn that hospitalization is required. Otherwise sensible people have been known to do things like fall asleep under the lamp, miscalculate the distance between the bulb and their face, forget to put on the all-important goggles, etc.

In order to use a sunlamp properly, you will need:
1. the lamp itself
2. a timer (5 seconds is considered a reasonable first exposure time)
3. goggles (sunglasses are *not* sufficient protection)
4. a sunscreen

There are three types of sunlamps that you're likely to encounter. The first and most common has a screw-in reflector bulb. At the moment, most bulbs can fit in the average household socket. It should be noted that the extreme heat generated by this bulb can sometimes melt an ordinary socket. So, testing is highly advisable.

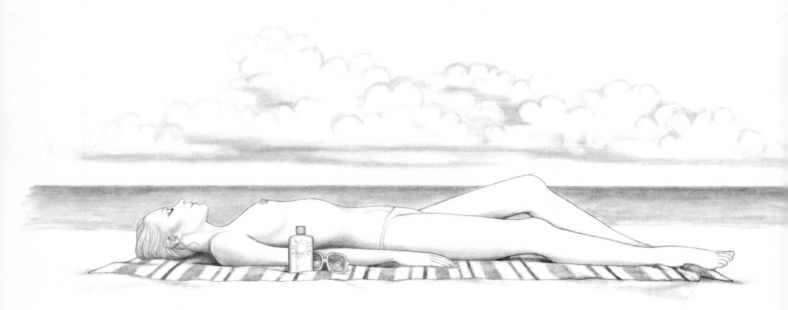

The fluorescent bulb is next in popularity and often encountered in health spas. Like the reflector bulb, it is constructed of specially treated glass that encloses mercury vapor.

The third type of sunlamp comes with a metal reflector and often includes both an infrared and an incandescent light. The type of glass used does not filter out short-wavelength ultraviolet radiation, which makes it the most dangerous.

In the future, thanks to FDA rulings, you will be unable to buy lamps without proper housings, goggles, and built-in timers. But until those rulings take effect, it's up to you to get all the separate items you'll need.

Frankly, sunlamp tanning should not be undertaken unless you're blessed with lots and lots of stick-to-it-iveness. Getting an even color is chancy, and the danger of bad burns is a constant threat. No sunlamp is a satisfactory substitute for natural sunlight in terms of the quality of the color you can expect to get. You have to have a "touch" for good results—that is, you must find exactly the right "dosage" of sunlamp time, exactly the right frequency of sunlamp sessions, and maintain the optimum distance from the sunlamp. And it's a "touch" that not everybody has.

INSTANT TANNING

A variety of products on the market promise instant, or sunless, tans. The chemical tan, which affects only the top layer of skin, is induced by means of a chemical called dihydroxyacetone (DHA). Assuming you're not allergic to DHA, the instant tanners are safe enough, even though some critics maintain that no one would mistake a chemical tan for the genuine article. Only trial and error will determine just how good a DHA tan looks on your skin. Of course, what looks artificial under the harsh light of noon will undoubtedly seem much more natural in a disco at midnight.

Whatever you do at midnight, don't assume that because you look tanned, you can therefore race out into the noon sun with no protection. Only a few of the quick tanning products contain sunscreens, and unless you've built up protection from the lower layers of skin, you'll still risk a bad burn.

Successful use of DHA products takes patience and consistency. Directions usually suggest two or three applications, applied as soon as the preceding layer is dry. When too casually applied, the resulting "tan" can look streaky. Sometimes it turns orange on certain skin types. And it will stay that way until it wears off—maybe days or even weeks later.

Devotees rely on these products for the illusion of a tanned leg when it's really too early in the season to have a suntan, but warm enough to want to be free of pantyhose. Another use is as strap-mark fillers when the bodice of an evening dress doesn't gibe with that of your swimsuit. It's usually only a matter of hours between application and final results.

If you're simply interested in a short-term "fake" tan until you can get the real thing, it might be a better idea to try one of the cosmetic bronzers that do not contain DHA. They are translucent, easily applied, and give a sort of glow that the DHA tanners lack. Application requires gently massaging the bronzer onto the skin at reasonable speed, since bronzers dry quickly. And, if you don't like the effect, it's easy to wash off immediately with soap and water. Bronzers are available in gel and stick form, the former being easier to apply, at least in our opinion.

Remember: Whenever using DHA or bronzers, always wash your hands *very thoroughly* after application. Stained palms are not chic.

COPING WITH SUNBURN

Despite all our admonitions you stayed out on the beach too long, or dozed off briefly under the sunlamp, and the result was a sunburn. What should you do?

If it's a mild sunburn, take an aspirin or two (unless nauseated) and slip into a tepid tub, to which you've added 2 cups of either cider vinegar or bicarbonate of soda. Lie still for 20 minutes, making sure all the affected areas are submerged, and add hot water as the tub cools so as to keep the temperature constant. Two and one-quarter cups of laundry starch or the same amount of uncooked oatmeal are acceptable soothing alternatives to the vinegar or the bicarbonate of soda.

On leaving the tub, gently pat yourself dry. Then apply a commercial sunburn palliative or any product containing benzocaine, a mild topical anaesthetic. If you're allergic to benzocaine, any moisturizer will make an acceptable second choice. Lacking that, you can turn to the kitchen cabinet and try vegetable oil.

Unfortunately, no amount of tender loving care will prevent peeling. The severity of the burn has already determined how extensive that peeling will be. The process can continue for as long as two weeks, and no matter how great the temptation, *do not* sunbathe during that time. The result can be a mottled tan that may even linger on as mottled skin long after the tan fades.

Of course, if you're in extreme discomfort, nauseated, or see blisters beginning to form, go to a doctor. A second-degree burn can take the form of fever, chills, even vomiting or delirium. No drugstore preparation or home-grown formula is going to offer much relief, and with a severe burn of any kind, there is always the possibility of infection.

We'll close this chapter with a sober observation. You must invariably lose when and if you try to cut corners in tanning. With so many good sunscreens and sunblocks on the market, you have only yourself to blame for a sunburn. Not only is that burn a problem in itself, it will also compel you either to stay indoors until it heals, or risk looking as if you have some peculiar skin disease for a long time to come. So play it safe and take it slow.

2. You and the Sun: The Medical View

Sunlight, or natural light, is just a tiny fraction of the total energy given off by the sun. This total energy is also called radiant energy, or electromagnetic energy, and it moves toward Earth in waves of different lengths, depending upon how much energy the waves carry. For our health—and our tans—the most important types of radiant energy are ultraviolet rays, visible light rays, and infrared rays.

VISIBLE LIGHT

You've probably seen a prism or a rainbow separate light into its component parts—the visible-light spectrum. There are actually over 100 colors in this spectrum, but the major bands (the colors of the rainbow) are red, orange, yellow, green, blue, indigo, and violet light—in that order, from longest to shortest wavelength. Scientists measure the wavelengths of all radiant energy in units called Angstroms (A). The wavelengths of visible light range from about 4300A on the short, violet end, to about 6800A on the long, red end.

INVISIBLE LIGHT

Surrounding the visible light spectrum on either side are the two kinds of invisible light—infrared and ultraviolet. Infrared rays have wavelengths longer than those of red. They are, very simply, heat rays, whose sole purpose is to make things hot. Ultraviolet energy, with wavelengths shorter than violet light, are another matter entirely. Their known effects on the human body are numerous, and we're still learning new things about them. Most of what we've heard to date about ultraviolet (UV) has been bad. But new findings give a more balanced picture.

Sunlight reflected off water (or snow) can increase your chance of getting burned.

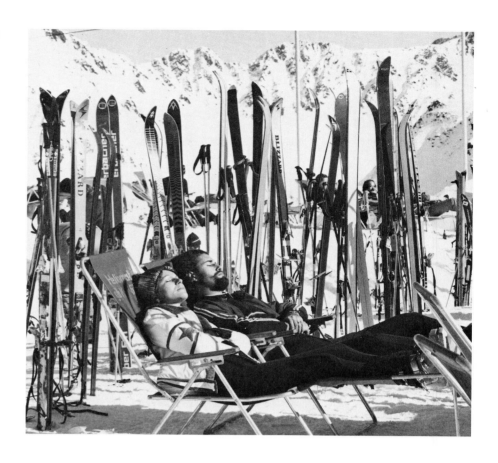

ULTRAVIOLET LIGHT

There are really three kinds of UV light, which are commonly referred to as UVA, UVB, and UVC. The variety with the shortest wavelength, UVC, is also know as germicidal light, so called because germs exposed to UVC die. Most natural UVC is filtered out by the Earth's ozone layer, so that very little of it ever reaches us down below. That's why many thinking people are concerned about ozone destruction by aerosol sprays and supersonic aircraft. UVC is dangerous: It can destroy human tissue and other living things.

The other two varieties of UV are far safer and far more controllable. UVA rays, the longest of the UV rays, have a wavelength range of 3200–4000A. They are, among other things, the rays that *tan* us. UVBs, the middle-length UVs, have wavelengths from 2900–3200A: They are the rays that *burn* us. Yes, tanning and burning rays are different, which should clear up one very common misconception: *You don't have to burn in order to tan.* All you have to do is control the UVs, allowing the tanning As to penetrate the skin, while blocking out the burning Bs.

UV, and particularly UVB, is certainly involved in a broad range of potential hazards to our health and well-being. But the evidence continues to mount that the UV reaching us in natural sunlight has widespread positive effects on our bodies as well, and that a lack of UV can actually be unhealthy. As a cause

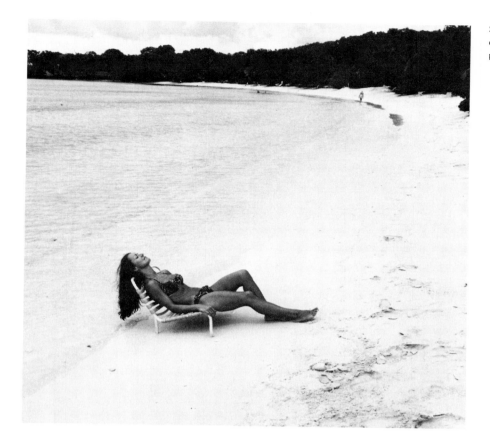

Sun has beneficial effects: it stimulates our sex hormones and enhances vitamin D production.

of skin cancer, for example, UV may not be as nasty a villain as we had once thought.

FULL-SPECTRUM LIGHT

When light contains both visible and invisible wavelengths, we call it "full-spectrum." Sunlight is full-spectrum light. Most artificial light, invented by man simply to overcome darkness, isn't full-spectrum. Incandescent bulbs and fluorescent tubes are the prevalent forms of artificial light. Both radiate plenty of visible light and plenty of infrared (heat), but neither provides any UVs to speak of. Since most window glass filters the UVs out of natural sunlight, the result is that many of us receive very little full-spectrum light. However, some recent research indicates that such light—which contains UVs—has benefits for us that are only beginning to be understood. Many experts now believe that certain metabolic disorders are the result of insufficient natural, full-spectrum light, and that UVA in particular has therapeutic effects on many diseases, including psoriasis, arthritis, and cancer.

Various laboratory tests and on-site studies suggest the possibility that UV-inclusive light helps workers reduce fatigue and accidents and dramatically increases productivity. It also appears to decrease susceptibility to colds and helps absorb calcium from food. Doctors have known for some time that UV acts as a catalyst on certain skin secretions, transforming them to natural vitamin D, which is then absorbed into the bloodstream. Vitamin D is in itself an important nutrient and is also crucial to our utilization of calcium and phosphorus.

A great deal of fascinating research now surrounds the effect of light on the hormone-producing glands of the human endocrine system. These studies have demonstrated that UV-inclusive, full-spectrum light has effects on certain endocrine-related biochemical processes and disease patterns different from those of pure visible light. This discovery holds the promise of possible breakthroughs in our understanding of medical problems as diverse as diabetes, cancer, and infertility. Last but not least, experiments at various medical research centers have begun to produce solid evidence that light containing UVs stimulates growth and activity of the sex organs and enhances human sexual response.

Light that has a direct impact on delicate hormonal balances enters through the eyes, sending certain hormone levels up, others down. Since it's also become apparent that individual chemical balances are affected by specific wavelengths of light entering the system, it's easy to see why anything you put between your eyes and natural light is going to change the light's energy characteristics and influence these levels. Window glass and plain corrective lenses filter the UVs out of natural light, artificial light doesn't have UVs to begin with, and sunglasses filter not only UVs, but certain colors of visible light as well. Blindness, of course, often means that no light energy is transmitted by the eye, and it's significant that most blind people have highly irregular endocrine rhythms.

All of this is not to suggest that UV is some kind of panacea or to deny its well-documented ability to cause medical problems, particularly for the skin. But we might do well to plan our exposure to UV, to be sensible about it, rather than to simply eliminate it altogether.

There are some fairly simple steps you can take to increase your exposure to light containing UVs. Full-spectrum fluorescent tubes are available and so is window glass that transmits UVs and material for both clear corrective lenses and even sunglasses. In short, don't close your eyes to the benefits of natural, full-spectrum light.

THE SUN AND YOUR SKIN

The skin is your body's barrier against the outside world, and it takes a lot of punishment while trying to protect the rest of you from harm. Much of this punishment comes at the hands of the sun, whose rays could otherwise cause tremendous damage to delicate body chemistry. Tanning is a natural response to protect the body from excess UVB exposure. When you help your skin to tan safely and thoroughly, you're actually helping it to guard against many far more damaging effects of the sun. In the simplest sense, a suntan is the result of a UVA-stimulated increase in production and distribution of melanin. It's helpful to tan yourself carefully because melanin, our natural sunscreen, is probably the most effective one around.

Skin is divided into two main compartments—the epidermis, or outer layer, and the dermis beneath it. Your skin contains one-third of all the blood circulating in your body. If you're average sized—say about 5'5", 120 lbs.—your skin's surface area is a bit over 3000 square inches, and it accounts for at least 6 percent of your total weight—a little over 7 pounds. It's very flexible, and some

Sunhats offer tender skin protection from the burning effects of ultra-violet rays.

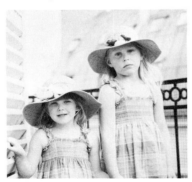

20

skin areas can stretch for a few seconds by as much as 50 percent and return to normal almost immediately. Skin thickness varies from one person to the next and from spot to spot, but an average range would be from 1/32 inch on the eyelids, to 1/8 inch on the upper back.

One square centimeter (.39 square inches) of skin contains approximately:

15 sebaceous glands
100 sweat glands
1 yard of blood vessels
12 nerves
10 hairs
3000 sensory cells at nerve-fiber ends
200 nerve endings to record pain
25 pressure receptors for touch stimuli
12 sensory receptors for heat
2 sensory receptors for cold
3,000,000 cells

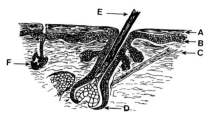

The skin is the largest organ in the human body. Composed of millions of constantly rejuvenating cells—it is divided into layers: the outer epidermis (A) and the basilar layer (B) are the body's first line of defense against sun, wind, and cold. The nerve fibrils (C) generate our very developed sense of touch. Hair follicles (D) produce hair shafts (E) that puncture the epidermis, and oil glands (F) lubricate the skin.

The epidermis. The skin that meets the eye, figuratively speaking, is the top layer of epidermis—the stratum corneum, or horny layer. The most intriguing characteristic of this skin is that it's dead. Millions of horny layer cells disappear from your body daily; they are washed, rubbed, or burned away. When you're tan, these dead surface cells contain much of your visible melanin. So, if you think you've lost a little of your tan in the shower, you have—down the drain. But on the bright side, one flight below, at the basal or Malpighian level, your skin can be at work producing more.

The Malpighian level is the bottom layer of epidermis. It's comprised of round basal cells, flatter squamous cells, and the melanin-producing cells called melanocytes. New epidermal cells are manufactured here to replace those lost each day and are slowly pushed up to the surface by the even newer cells behind them. On average, your epidermis is completely renewed every fifteen days—roughly the time it takes new cells to complete the trip from lower Malpighian to upper horny layer.

The dermis. Below the epidermis is the more structurally complex dermis. Almost all of the skin's major chemical activity goes on here, with the exception of the melanin production upstairs in the epidermis. The dermis is home to sweat and oil glands, blood vessels, hair follicles, nerves, and other less well-known components. Of these, among the most important for sun lovers are those cells that produce the proteins called collagen and elastin. Together, these proteins comprise the elastic tissue that gives skin suppleness, tone, and resiliency. When this tissue is weakened or damaged, it results in wrinkling, sagging, and other signs of aging.

Damage to the elastic tissue and to various cell processes of the dermis is caused by UVBs. The epidermis works to prevent such damage in two ways—by thickening, and by melanin production. Both occur spontaneously with increased sun exposure.

Put on your bikini, throw a towel over your shoulder, and stroll down to your favorite sun spot. Unless you do something to interfere, the sun can tan or burn you with equal ease. However, with a few facts and some common sense (unless you're one of the unlucky few who have no sun tolerance at all)

The skin surface (A) is constantly rejuvenated by the production of new cells (B), softened by oil (C) and cooled by perspiration glands (D).

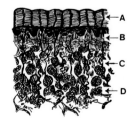

you can opt for a tan every time. Remember that tanning and burning are two entirely different processes. Today's tan can prevent tomorrow's burn.

ANATOMY OF A SUNTAN

Tanning rays are UVAs at wavelengths in the 3200–4000A range. These rays trigger increases in both production and dispersion of the tanning pigment, melanin. The melanocytes in the basal layer produce melanin granules, which are automatically distributed among all living cells in the epidermis. In the untanned state, these granules have a tendency to congregate within each cell, to varying degrees most likely determined by heredity. Albinos have no melanin at all. Blacks, on the other hand, generally have about the same amount of melanin as Caucasians, but the melanin granules are more widely dispersed within each cell, creating a darker overall appearance. Think of two glasses of water side by side, each with a drop of india ink placed carefully on top. Stir one of the glasses, and it will end up looking darker, although it contains no more ink than its neighbor. UVAs stir the melanin in our cells. The longer the exposure, the greater stirring, or dispersion, of the granules within each cell. The tanning rays also trigger an actual increase in the number of melanin-producing cells. They also trigger an increase in their production of new granules, which are first distributed among the cells, then dispersed within them. The combined effect of more melanocytes, more granules, more dispersion, and the upward migration of these richly pigmented cells from basal to horny layer creates an increasingly dark tan.

ANATOMY OF A SUNBURN

A sunburn is a local skin injury caused by excessive exposure to UVBs. While the entire part of the UVB range from 2900–3100A can burn you, the most powerful burn rays are in the even narrower band from 3050–3080A.

When less is more—as in a bikini—you want to tan, not burn.

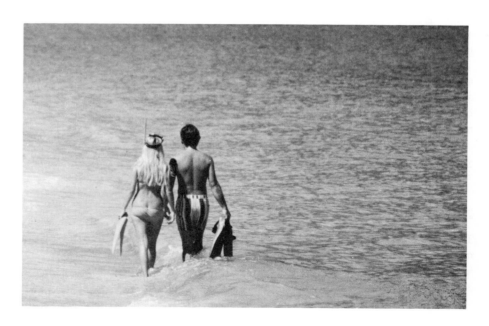

The UVBs start several chains of events that combine to create the redness, pain, and swelling of a sunburn. One major assault begins in the epidermal cells, where the burning rays cause tiny enzyme packets, called lysosomes, to burst. Every cell has a lysosome. It's a built-in self-destructing capsule. When it bursts, it destroys the cell and releases its irritating enzymes into the surrounding tissue. The blood vessels near the top of the dermis are the burn rays' second major point of attack. The UVBs cause these vessels to dilate, or enlarge, and more blood flows through the dilated vessels. The enlargement is typically accompanied by a freeing of chemicals in the skin that cause the walls of the vessels to leak. They leak a combination of clear liquid, called serum or edema fluid, and blood toxins—impurities that would otherwise be filtered out of the bloodstream by the kidneys, liver, and other excretory organs.

When the toxins leak into the skin, they further the irritating effect of released lysosome enzymes, and together they cause redness (erythema) and pain. The leaked serum creates blistering and swelling (edema). Redness, pain, swelling, blistering—sunburn.

Tanning can help save you from all that, by blocking many of the UVBs. At the same time, a tan can counter oily skin, and guard against solar elastosis—damage to the elastic tissue—with its attendant wrinkling, sagging, and atrophy of the skin. While you're best off supplementing it with a good commercial sunscreen, a tan is a smart investment.

SUNBURNS: SIGNS, SYMPTOMS, AND SIZING UP THE SITUATION

If you're lying on the beach and think you're burning, you probably are. If you've been basking unprotected in the noonday sun for a half hour or more, you're probably burning even if you *don't* think so. A severe sunburn can bring chills, fever, kidney inflammation, vomiting, and delirium. It also produces serious blistering that might become infected and then scar. Don't tell yourself that the redness you're seeing and the discomfort you're feeling will pass. It won't. And if you *do* become badly burned, get medical attention. It's far better, though, to arm yourself. Take the necessary precautions—burning is not a prerequisite to a suntan.

Developing a feel for your personal sun tolerance, and evaluating the probable intensity of the UVs that will confront you where and when you plan to sunbathe, are two basic techniques of smart sunning. The other items in your bag of precautionary tricks will depend on the results of these two measurements. The conditions affecting UV intensity, discussed in the previous chapter, include the date, the time of day, the weather, the physical environment, and geography. Here are some pointers to help you evaluate your personal tolerance for sun-exposure.

HOW THE SUN STRIKES YOU

The first overt sign of a sunburn is an initial faint redness, medically called mild erythema. It's often accompanied by a slight tingling discomfort, resulting from the first release of chemical irritants in the skin. The length of exposure necessary to produce that initial redness in *unprotected* skin is known as the Minimum Erythemal Dose, or MED. While the actual MED will vary with the intensity of UVBs, and this, in turn, will vary with specific circumstances, some average MEDs have been determined for noonday summer sun on a clear day, at a location midway between the equator and the poles. They are 15 minutes for fair skin, 20 minutes for average skin, and 25 minutes for dark skin.

The mild erythema disappears quickly, but 2 to 6 hours later redness returns, far brighter now and with considerable skin tenderness. The peak of the pain, redness, and swelling from sunburn is generally reached after 15 to 24 hours, but symptoms may last up to 72 hours.

Once you pass your MED, you're probably in for all the symptoms of a mild burn—skin that's hot, red, taut, and tender to the touch. At this point, getting out of the sun will be the only really intelligent choice open to you. Remaining unprotected in the sun anywhere from three to nine or ten times your MED will produce a moderate to severe burn, depending upon your pigmentation.

But you can avoid the problem altogether by applying an effective sunscreen at the outset. The most effective screens for tanning, such as those containing 5 percent PABA in an alcohol base, will filter out most of the burning UVBs, but not the tanning UVAs. Sunscreens *don't make you tan faster.* In fact, for the same amount of sun, a sunscreen often makes you tan a bit more slowly. But you won't be limited to the same amount of sun. You'll be able to tolerate far *more* sun, safely, without burning. A good sunscreen multiplies your MED by eight times or more, so you can work on your tan far longer each day.

Skin thickness will also affect your MED, and thickness increases naturally with sun exposure over time. Age can be a factor as well. Infants tend to be extremely sensitive to sun, so keep the baby covered up on the beach. The elderly have fewer melanocytes, and sometimes the remaining ones lose their ability to produce new pigment. On the other hand, most people's skin darkens a bit with age, the result of a spontaneous increase in melanin dispersion. Where the balance will fall is hard to predict, so it's best to be cautious.

Sun, sand, and sweat can irritate tender skin.

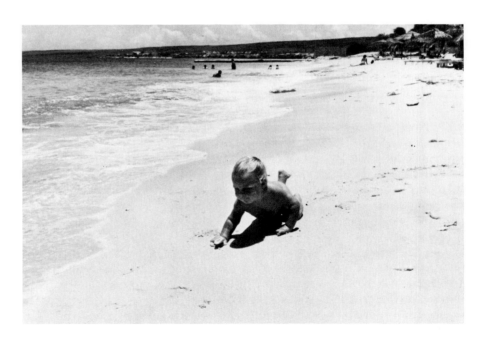

AN OUNCE OF PREVENTION

Once you've sized up your skin and the situation, you can make all the right moves to avoid solar misery. Your most sensible sunburn protection will be the combination of a good sunscreen and a tan, unless your skin is so sensitive that it requires the total UVA and UVB filtering provided by a true sunblock. There are physical sunblocks, like zinc oxide paste, and chemical ones, like lotions containing both benzophenones and UVB filters. Sunblocks screen out everything, including UVAs, so you won't tan with a sunblock. But they're necessary to protect small areas of sunburned skin, like your nose or shoulders, from continued exposure while you're trying to tan the rest of you.

Even if you're fair skinned, you can probably get some tan by repeated small doses of UVAs. Since there's a limit to the amount of melanin your body can produce, you may never get a dark tan, but every little bit helps. Keep in mind, though, that even the most effective sunscreens only shield us from about 85 percent of the UVBs. Not even melanin blocks out all the UVBs, and the damage they do to the tissues is almost all *cumulative*. It occurs quite slowly, gets a little worse with each exposure, and never repairs itself. Keep your UVB exposure to a minimum by using sunscreens *all the time*.

Plain oils and moisturizers are almost useless for preventing sunburns. Mineral oil or baby oil, for instance, used alone or mixed with iodine, will neither prevent a burn nor promote a tan. Their moisturizing effect is negligible, since you can't really seal in moisture during a sunbath. In fact, excessive grease in heavy oils can clog your pores and lead to pimples. It can also combine with the effects of sweating and the sun's general irritation of the skin to produce an itchy rash and/or inflammed hair follicles (follicilitis).

Clothes, of course, will provide solid protection from further UV exposure once you've decided to call it a day. If you're burned, loose clothes will minimize the discomfort from friction. Generally, nonporous clothes block more UVs. Broad-brimmed hats and long sleeves make sense, even gloves in extreme cases. Regarding color, the most effective protection is offered by a combination of a light layer over a dark one. The light layer will reflect most of the UVs away, while the dark bottom layer will absorb those that do get through.

COPING WITH SUNBURN

If you have somehow managed to get a sunburn despite all this good advice, vow to make it your last one, and minimize your suffering for the day or two that you must bear with it. If you've gotten a severe burn, take a few aspirin and call a doctor. You can treat a mild burn, cautiously, on your own. There's no one approach that is best suited for everyone, but most successful home regimens contain many or all of the following steps:

1. Short cool baths: Post-sun hydration can make the burn less damaging and drying to your skin. Take a cool bath with some oil in it for five or ten minutes. Pat yourself dry, and apply a urea moisturizer.

2. Application of wet compresses: These relieve pain by drawing heat out of the burn. Two formulas come highly recommended. *Formula 1:* add a tablespoon of salt and six ounces of skim milk to a quart container filled with crushed ice. *Formula 2:* To two quarts of cool water or milk add one tablespoon

each of cornstarch and baking soda. In either case, dip a gauze or cloth in the mixture and apply it to the burn for ten or fifteen minutes. You can also try a simple paste of baking soda and water. Apply it, let it dry, and rinse it off.

3. Use of soothing lotions, creams, or ointments: Baby lotion, petroleum jelly, and cold cream are all somewhat soothing. Avoid drying lotions, like calamine. Try some talcum powder between your sheets.

4. Aspirin: This will reduce the discomfort, unless you're allergic to it.

5. Commercial sunburn remedies: Most of these, whether ointments or sprays, contain both an oil to lubricate burned tissue and a topical anesthetic to deaden surface nerve endings. Benzocaine and its chemical relatives are the most popular pain killers, but benzocaine causes allergic responses in some people, which can lead to a rash on top of the burn! If this double disaster should strike you, don't bother trying other benzocaine products. If you're allergic to one, you will be allergic to all. Cautiously, you might try a product containing lidocaine or dibucaine. Otherwise, a camphorated lotion should give you some relief.

6. Stay out of the sun: A rule that should be followed in every sound sunburn-treatment regimen. Burned skin generally takes two or three weeks to return to normal.

A final truth about sunburns—they peel, and there's nothing you can do to prevent it. If you're burned, you've got blisters, even if they're too small to see with the naked eye. Blisters are the result of skin traumas that pull the dermis and epidermis apart. During the sunburn trauma, they fill with the edema fluid that leaks out of dilated blood vessels. Once the fluid drains and the swelling goes down, the dead skin on top is going to shed. That's peeling, and it can't be stopped or even delayed. In dry climates, a moisturizer will minimize the tight, prickly feeling of your burn; but it won't prevent peeling—nothing will.

THE SUN AND SKIN CANCER

The sun burns millions of people every year. But if you asked the average sunbather what, if anything, concerns her about the sun, the likely reply would be "skin cancer." Back in the days when ladies wore bustles and carried parasols, 4 out of 5 skin cancers appeared in men. Today, it's about half and half. While most occur in people over 50, there's been a significant increase among the 22 to 35 age group, especially women. Malignancies are rare before the twenties. However, since the UVB exposure that contributes to skin cancer is cumulative, significant damage can be built up by the late teens, which will only become cancerous sometime later.

Light-skinned, blue-eyed people with a family history of skin cancers are statistically the most likely to develop them, which suggests some hereditary connection. In fact, in one survey of skin cancer patients at a Chicago hospital clinic, 46 percent were either born in Ireland or of Irish extraction.

All tumors and lesions are abnormal growths. But if they remain controlled, if they neither spread nor invade surrounding tissues, they're *benign* and not cancerous. Many strange-looking skin lesions, particularly on elderly people, are merely such benign, noncancerous growths. If a growth is uncontrolled, however, its cells will produce new tissues for unknown reasons. Such growths choke out normal tissues and extend to adjacent tissue layers. Uncontrolled growths are called malignant, or cancerous.

Like other malignancies, those on the skin grow in three ways—either by expansion (spreading on the skin), invasion (growing down through the dermis), or by metastasis (spreading to other sites within the body). Cancers of any variety are very rarely terminal unless they metastasize—in which case they are always fatal eventually. Skin cancers are rarely fatal because they rarely metastasize. Most skin cancers don't even *look* frightening—rather like a brownish discoloration, or a case of acne.

The three types of skin cancer. The total number of all new cancers, or carcinomas, in the United States is approaching 1,000,000 annually. Of these, about one-third are skin cancers. While skin cancers cause 7,000 deaths annually, this represents only 2 percent of all cancer deaths. There are three types of skin cancer—basal cell carcinoma, squamous cell carcinoma, and malignant melanoma. Almost all of the deaths from skin cancer are due to the melanomas. That's because, with few exceptions, melanomas are the only skin cancers that metastasize. They are, fortunately, also very rare. The National Cancer Institute puts the total number of new basal and squamous cell carcinomas in the United States at over 300,000 per year, with a five-year survival rate of over 95 percent. The number of new melanomas annually is 9,000. While your prognosis is far shakier if you've got a melanoma, the survival rate for even this potentially lethal malignancy is almost 65 percent.

The sun is clearly implicated as a contributing cause to all skin cancers—to one degree or another. But increasingly, researchers are questioning the degree. Almost all specialists now believe that certain other factors beside UVs are involved, particularly with respect to basal carcinomas.

Considerable attention is now focusing on the genetic material DNA and its possible role in causing cancer. Solar radiation is believed to damage the DNA in the nuclei of epidermal cells. Under normal conditions, cell mechanisms automatically repair the sun-damaged DNA. One hypothesis suggests that this repair system can malfunction for reasons that may have nothing to do with the sun, and that the unrepaired DNA stimulates the abnormal cancerous growth.

Certainly, skin cancers are the most frightening and most serious of the sun-related skin problems, but the reality is that they are the mildest, least dangerous cancers around. They often share little with their deadlier cousins beyond the family name. The overall cure rate for skin cancers is now about 95 percent, and many doctors think we could eliminate fatalities completely if people would seek treatment early enough.

OTHER SUN AND SKIN PROBLEMS

Not content with sunburns and cancer, the sun displays distressing ingenuity in getting under our skin, which, in turn, displays a distressing array of spots, sags, wrinkles, and rashes. Most of these can be kept under control, however, with some care, caution, common sense, and a good dermatologist.

While it's generally accepted that UVAs have no particular aging effect on the skin, UVBs are known to have cumulative damaging results. A lifetime of exposure can leave you with leathery skin that's wrinkled, sagging, dry, perhaps even scarred. Crow's feet have been traced to sun damage, and all wrinkles look more pronounced on sun-damaged areas.

Wrinkles, sags, and droops. UVBs slowly alter the skin's elastic supportive tissues, comprised of collagen and elastin, which give skin tone and resiliency. Destruction of collagen produces wrinkles; damage to elastin leads to sagging or drooping. Neither locally applied hormones nor cosmetics containing collagen are of any help in reversing the damage. But it can be repaired by application of a truly miraculous drug called topical 5-fluorouracil ointment, which has the astonishing ability to selectively destroy damaged tissue, leaving the healthy surrounding tissue alone. What's more, it will also excise tissues that look fine now, but will start to show their damage five years from now. Treatment with 5-fluorouracil can eliminate future cancers, too. Treatment is not very painful, nor is it pleasant; typically, it lasts 2 to 3 months and eventually restores even skin tone.

Liver spots. Years of exposure to sun and wind cause the common, dark, irregular patches known as liver spots, age spots, or senile lentigo. Such spots, which have nothing to do with the liver, most often appear on the face, backs of hands and arms, and lower legs. They can be removed by acids or electric needles, but it's difficult since they're not raised. They're very rarely dangerous, however, so they can probably safely be left alone.

Freckles. Freckles are the result of uneven melanin dispersion, so it's quite logical that they'll get even darker in the sun. Since the darkening is caused by UVAs, most sunscreens won't help. Try one of the UVA screens containing benzophenones, but mix it with a UVB screen so you won't burn.

The freckle problem, if you consider it one, begins in the melanocytes, and appears to be genetically determined. Bleaches containing hydroquinone may lighten freckles, but you must avoid the sun while using them, and they usually take months or years before producing results, if any.

The sun and pregnancy. Your skin is essentially unchanged during pregnancy. But various pigmented bodies—moles, freckles, and birthmarks—tend to become darker spontaneously. This is caused by excess melanin production stimulated by the high levels of estrogen circulating in your system. Cloasma, the "mask of pregnancy," may also develop, in the form of dark blotches on the forehead, cheeks, abdomen, or elsewhere. Cloasma (sometimes called melasma) is accentuated by sunlight, and it's most common in brunettes and other dark-complected women. Use of a sunblock, or a benzophenone sunscreen, can help to minimize the darkening. Otherwise, try a wide-brimmed hat.

Both genital herpes simplex and the oral variety, commonly called a fever blister, can be activated by the sun. Genital herpes is a particular threat to pregnant women, as it can infect the fetus during delivery and produce birth defects or fetal death. Be sure to advise your obstetrician if you suspect you've contracted herpes during your term.

The sun and the pill. Birth control pills, both the estrogen and progesterone types, can produce "artificial" cloasma. The melanocytes appear to be stimulated by the hormones in oral contraceptives, and the excess melanin creates blotches that often take months to go away, and they are sometimes permanent. You must avoid the sun, or use UVA screens or blocks if cloasma appears. Some dermatologists recommend taking the pill at night, so that the hormone levels will be at their lowest during the hours of sun exposure.

In addition to cloasma, the pill occasionally causes the rare syndrome called porphyria, in which sunlight transforms skin chemicals into toxic agents that produce itching, burning and swelling. Regular doses of carotene (vitamin A) in pill form can keep porphyria under control. A final caution about the pill: Like many other substances, it can produce unpleasant photosensitive reactions.

Photosensitivity. "Sun poisoning" is a layman's term for a wide variety of fleeting or enduring skin conditions that are known to doctors as photosensitivities. All such skin reactions require the presence of a sensitizing agent— and the sun.

Some photosensitizers simply increase the speed with which you'll get a bad burn. Others lead to inflamed, red, itchy areas, or rashes. Lightening or darkening of the affected spots sometimes persists long after the more immediate symptoms have gone.

Photosensitivities can be triggered by light wavelengths between 2800 and 4000A. That means both UVAs and UVBs. A few reactions can even be set off by the light coming through ordinary window glass, or from fluorescent tubes. Specific photosensitive agents respond to specific wavelengths of light. So, if you use a photosensitizer either before or during sun exposure, you could have a problem.

Photosensitivity can be broken down into two broad categories of response —phototoxicity and photoallergy. Phototoxicity can strike anyone, given sufficient doses of both a phototoxic agent and sunlight. The typical response is characterized by a tingling, burning, itching sensation, often with redness and swelling. The reaction is limited to sun-exposed parts of the body and will develop after anywhere from a few minutes to several hours of sun exposure. The response almost always stops, however, when you discontinue use of the phototoxic agent.

Photoallergies, which are less common, only strike certain people, and may be genetically determined. They can appear on both sun-exposed and protected areas and are usually delayed. Typically, the reactions appear from 5 to 7 days after one sun exposure, and are set off by a reexposure. The degree of response is often unrelated to the doses of sun and allergen, and the allergies can persist, sometimes for months or years, after the agent has been eliminated.

The enemies list. There are lots of photosensitizers, and a few of the more common troublemakers may come as unpleasant surprises.

Diet soft drinks contain artificial sweeteners (including saccharin) that are photosensitive and can lead to a nasty burn for some people who drink them during a sunbath. They can also cause blotchy dark spots that are sometimes permanent.

Oil of bergamot, found in many perfumes, can cause berlock dermatitis, an irritation that often leaves permanent splotches around the neck and throat even after the blistering burns and rashes it produces have cleared up. Oils of rosemary and lavender, also found in some perfumes, can photosensitize, too.

Lime juice or essence found in some perfumes and aftershaves, can photosensitize from a random squirt as you prepare a cooling gin and tonic. It's *very* phototoxic, and belongs near the top of the list of potential hazards. Lemon juice, curiously, is not nearly as bad, though it is phototoxic.

Furocoumarins may not sound very common, but look again. These are toxic chemicals found in a family of foods that include not only limes, lemons, and bergamots, but also figs, parsnips, dill, fennel, parsley, carrots, and celery. These can be phototoxic if eaten or applied to the skin. The reaction depends on the dose.

Deodorant soaps often contain highly photosensitive chemicals called halogenated salicylanilides. Hotels in most sunny climates have stopped supplying rooms with deodorant soaps because of the sunburn danger.

Here's a list of some other common photosensitizers. Remember, some will respond to UVAs—tanning rays. Also, if the circumstances suggest a photoallergy, the problem stems from something you've used before, probably 5 to 10 days ago. With a little detective work, you and your dermatologist should be able to get the offender out of your life.

  birth control pills
  some antiseptic lotions and creams
  hexachlorophene
  some synthetic detergents
  some shampoos
  some hair conditioners
  some medicated cosmetics
  sulfonamides (used to treat bacterial infections)
  barbiturates
  some tranquilizers (e.g., thorazine)
  thiazide diuretics (water pills used to control high blood pressure)
  many hypoglycemics (oral diabetic drugs)
  griseofulvin (used to treat fungal infections)
  second generation tetracyclines (used to treat acne)
  analine dyes
  some anticonvulsive medicines
  certain sunscreens
  gold salts
  quinine and quinones (used to treat malaria)
  coal tars, wood tars, and some other fossil petroleum products (found in
    some cosmetics)

IF YOU CAN'T STAND THE HEAT . . .

UVs aren't the only rays that can cause problems on a sunny day. At the other end of the sunlight spectrum are infrared heat rays. Heat can make you miserable, and we're a long way from creating sunscreens with thermal barriers.

Your body works hard to maintain its normal temperature of 98.6° F. When the difference between your internal temperature and that of the surrounding air isn't great enough, normal heat loss isn't fast enough. As body temperature begins to rise, the blood triggers a mechanism in the brain that controls your cooling system. The blood vessels dilate to permit more blood to carry more heat toward the skin surface, and the sweat glands are activated.

When sweat comes into contact with heated skin, it evaporates, which pulls new, cooler air toward the skin surface. But when the humidity is too high, the sweat can't evaporate quickly enough, and your temperature-control system begins to back up with excess heat. Fainting is one possible result of insufficient heat loss. When the blood vessels dilate, blood pressure goes down. If it goes down too far, insufficient oxygen reaches the brain, and you keel over. Too much sweating, on the other hand, can produce dehydration and a dangerous loss of salt, and salt is essential for proper tissue maintenance.

Air conditioning. Air conditioners regulate both temperature and humidity. The ideal setting for an air conditioner is about 10 degrees lower than the outside air. This should permit normal heat loss easily, just under the point of sweating. While few air conditioners provide manual humidity controls, most people are most comfortable when the humidity is in the 40–50 percent range. Air conditioners make the body's temperature-regulation work easier, and are clearly useful when extremes of heat and humidity strain our energy supplies. But excessive reliance on them can lower your resistance to infection, make you sluggish and lazy, and increase the likelihood of catching colds.

Humidity. High humidity can affect your moods. The damp, soggy sensation it produces can lead to listlessness, lethargy, even depression. But this can be a blessing in disguise, a built-in safeguard against the overexertions that can really let the heat get to you. From the mildest to the most debilitating heat-produced conditions: heat rash, heat prostration, heat cramps, and sunstroke.

Heat rash. Heat rash, also called prickly heat and miliaria, is a red, itchy eruption caused by a blockage of the sweat duct openings. In the body's attempt to push the sweat out, the walls of the ducts can rupture, causing an inflammation, or blisters. Thick coatings of suntan oil can aggravate the condition, as can the continued contact of warm, sweaty clothes sticking to the body.

Miliaria tends to break out where skin surfaces are close together, so it often appears in the skin folds of the overweight and, of course, infants. The best treatment is to dry it up. Calamine lotion generally does this quickly, and it can be supplemented by cool showers, dusting powders, air conditioning, and loose, light clothing. If you're prone to prickly heat, avoid excessive sweating and keep your skin cool and dry.

Heat prostration. Heat prostration, exhaustion, or collapse is your body's way of telling you it's losing too much water and salt. It alerts you by slowing down all body processes. The possible symptoms of this metabolic brown-out

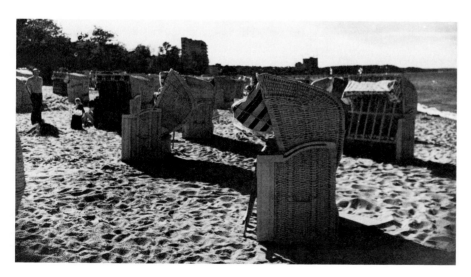

German sunbathers protect themselves from strong winds and sunburn with these mini-cabanas.

are headaches, palpitations, weak pulse, nausea, dizziness, weakness, blurred vision, mild muscle cramps, irritability, and pale, clammy skin.

Most victims only suffer some of these symptoms, but *all prostration victims sweat heavily.* This fact, along with their *moist skin* and *normal body temperature,* helps you to distinguish prostration victims from those of sunstroke (see below). Prostration, however, can degenerate into sunstroke if left untreated.

Victims of heat prostration should move to a cool environment, out of the sun. They should loosen their clothes, drink cool water, and replace lost salt.

You can avoid heat prostration by wearing light, loose clothing on hot days. Avoid overexertion, especially if it's humid. If you're sunbathing, take an occasional dip to cool off or spray yourself with cool water. Drink plenty of liquids, and take some extra salt with your food. Pretzels, potato chips, and other salty snacks are helpful.

Heat cramps. Heat cramps, also called stoker's cramps and fireman's cramps, are extremely painful. They're the result of salt loss from profuse sweating. Muscle cramps or spasms can grip the arms, legs, and sometimes the chest or abdomen. An attack of heat cramps strikes suddenly and can continue, intermittently, for hours if untreated. Victims often feel all right between spasms, but the cramps return with undiminished pain.

Victims should lie in a cool place and drink salt water—one teaspoon to a glass. The salt and water must be taken together, because drinking plain water first will simply dilute the body's remaining salt and make matters worse. Heat cramps call for medical attention. While waiting for the doctor, knotted muscles can be massaged and kneaded.

Guard against heat cramps by avoiding heavy work or exertion in extreme heat. If you must work, keep up your salt intake.

Sunstroke. Sunstroke, or heat stroke, kills 4,000 Americans every year. While 80 percent of the victims are over 50, sunstroke is the number-two cause of death among high school athletes. Needless to say, it's the most serious of the hot weather disorders.

Sunstroke results from the body's inability to cope with prolonged strenuous activity in extremes of heat. You must be acclimated to such exertions, and the U.S. Army estimates that it can take 4 to 6 weeks to build up significant heat tolerance. Your short vacation in the tropics won't do it.

When the body can't keep up with the accumulated heat, the brain's thermostat malfunctions, and body temperature soars out of control—typically to 106–107 degrees. The higher the fever, the greater the danger of irreversible tissue damage to the organs, particularly the heart, kidneys, and brain.

You don't even have to be out in the sun to suffer a heat stroke, but the risk is increased by intense sun, high humidity, poor ventilation, dehydration, heart disease, obesity, and especially alcoholism and advanced age.

Sunstroke can set in suddenly or gradually. It may start as a headache, dizziness, nausea, and weakness. Some victims show signs of apathy or confusion. The condition can deteriorate rapidly, first with the onset of muscle cramps, twitches, and delirium; eventually, coma, convulsions, and death.

A sunstroke victim has an extremely *rapid pulse,* and *hot, dry skin.* Most lose consciousness. The surest signs of sunstroke are *extreme fever* and *lack of sweating.* If you can't rush the victim to a hospital yourself, call an ambulance. In the meanwhile, the victim should be stripped, and either submerged in a cold bath or wrapped in cold wet sheets. Ice packs should be applied to head, arms, legs, and trunk. Fan the victim heavily, and try to restore lost salt and fluids. (Follow the heat cramp instructions given on page 32.) The cold wrappings should be kept on during the trip to the hospital. A cold tub or icepacks will generally bring body temperature back to normal in about 15 minutes. But most sunstroke victims must spend a few days in the hospital to recover fully. You can prevent sunstroke by avoiding overexertion and by diligently replacing the body fluids and salt lost through sweating.

OTHER CAUTIONS

Sun and wind. Wind seems to intensify most sun reactions, for reasons that aren't very clear. Perhaps it's because the cooling effects of wind disguise the actual amount of sun you're receiving. A strong wind, during skiing, for example, can cause the dry, scaly, or flaky skin condition called windburn. It's the result of dehydration, and it can be prevented by the liberal use of ointment that clings to the skin. Treat windburn by cooling down, moisturizing with oils or aftersun lotions, and cutting down on soaps.

Chapped lips are another result of dehydration from sun, wind, cold, or some combination of these elements. Glossy lipsticks offer good protection, but any physical barrier will do, like an ointment or zinc oxide paste, which should also be used to protect previously chapped lips against further dehydration.

Sun and salt water. Water dehydrates, with or without the sun, and salt water is even more drying. Although salt water doesn't reflect much sunlight—only about 5 percent—it does transmit light waves. So you can get a tan, or a burn, while swimming. Remember, too, that water will eventually wash off even the most binding sunscreens or blocks, so you'll only have whatever melanin you've built up to protect you. Reapply screens or blocks when you finish your dip.

The sun and your eyes. The great UV intensity at skiing altitudes can cause the itching inflammation called conjunctivitis, or pink-eye. The irritation is painful, but it can be cleared up quickly by your doctor. Goggles, which filter out most of the UVs, should prevent a recurrence.

Sunburned corneas, while extremely rare, are extraordinarily painful. If your eyes begin to sting from an intense glare, get out of the sun or put on sunglasses immediately. Some eclipse watchers, or others who contrive to stare at the sun, can contract solar retinitis, an inflammation of the part of the retina that receives the most distinct visual images. This is sunblindness, and it can be permanent.

A day in the sun can be a delight or a disaster. With some common sense, intuition, and the facts and explanations offered above, you'll develop a solid sun-sense. With it, you can step out onto your city rooftop, local beach, sun-drenched ski slope, or tropical paradise with increased chances of avoiding the disasters, and luxuriating in the delights.

3. Sunny Beauty: Your Face

For those who live in the Earth's temperate latitudes, the onset of summer signals a distinct change in the weather. Fortunately, it's a change for the better, at least for people who like spending time out of doors. Just as many of the simple rituals of daily living change to accommodate the warm weather, so skin care and makeup usually get their share of seasonal adjustment, too. Not everything changes, of course. In fact, quite a number of the sensible things one does to promote good skin and attractive looks remain constant throughout the year.

SKIN CARE

First, let's look briefly at summer skin care with an eye to what should and should not be altered for the season. Basically, the warm weather brings with it two important environmental changes: 1. humidity, and 2. increased sun exposure.

The increased humidity is good for almost everybody's skin. It helps ameliorate the discomforts associated with chronic dryness—things like tautness, dehydration-related wrinkling, and that stinging, pinprick feeling. Humidity naturally helps your moisturizer do its job more thoroughly, too, simply because it softens the dry winter environment that otherwise evaporates needed moisture from your skin's surface. For most normal skin types, then, the summertime humidity is simply a bonus that requires no alteration in one's personal care regimen.

As for sun exposure, which inevitably increases with the advent of summer, well, that's another story. Sun exposure, as we've already discussed, does very many good things. From a complexion standpoint, however, it must be handled with care. Possibly the best thing about sun exposure is its effect on the skin's cellular turnover rate. This, you'll recall, is the constant rate at which old cells are sloughed from the surface and replaced by plump new skin cells working their way up from below. A good turnover, or shed rate, is one that is fast enough to keep the pores unclogged, the complexion free of flakes, and the color of the skin clear and healthy. Sun exposure that allows a moderate amount of tanning—even if that tanning is barely perceptible—will help accomplish this.

However, this same amount of otherwise desirable sun exposure contains precisely those frequencies of ultraviolet light that contribute to premature aging. We bat the word "premature" around as if it were somehow natural to keep our skin in the dark forever. If we lived in caves, our skin would indeed appear less aged—but at a cost that is ridiculous to contemplate. We must accept a certain amount of sun-related aging as part of our lot in life. The name of the game is to limit it, and this can be accomplished effectively.

The best way to limit sun-related aging is *never* to go out in the sun without some sort of PABA protection. This advice is as valid in the winter as it is in the summer. And since you'll probably be out in the sun ten times as much in the summer, this advice about PABA is therefore ten times as important during the summer months. There are all sorts of ways to wear PABA. If you regularly use a foundation makeup, be sure it has PABA listed among the other ingredients. Fortunately, all cosmetic ingredients are now to be found somewhere on the packaging of every cosmetic marketed in the United States. If you don't wear foundation makeup, try to get whatever it is that you do use (blusher, highlighter, concealer, etc.) in a form containing PABA. You might also simply go to the drugstore and buy a little bottle of PABA gel or some similar pure PABA product, and scrupulously apply it whenever you're outdoors. In pure form, PABA is colorless and quite unnoticeable when dry. The protection it provides is invaluable. This advice is valid no matter what kind of skin you have.

WHAT'S RIGHT FOR YOUR SKIN TYPE?

This brings us to our next consideration—how to ascertain just what type of facial skin you really do have. The options aren't too extensive. Practically everybody's skin is either dry, oily, normal, or some combination thereof. What determines your skin type is the number of sebaceous oil glands you possess. Some people inherit these glands in abundance, others don't; it's purely a question of genetics. Sebaceous oil is the skin's own natural moisturizer, and its purpose is to retard the evaporation of surface moisture. This moisture is what keeps skin cells plump and smooth. Therefore, certain levels of oiliness are obviously quite desirable.

If you rub a piece of brown paper (of the supermarket bag variety) across your forehead and alongside your nose before washing in the morning, and that piece of paper becomes translucent, then your skin is of the oily variety—*too* oily, in fact. The brown paper test we've just described can warn you that your oil glands may literally clog up your own pores. This means you have to be extra careful with heavy makeups and moisturizers. Excessive oiliness is exactly what causes teenage acne—a condition we all know is not limited to teenagers. If you're an oily-skin type, you should welcome the summer tan. It will promote the peeling away of surface oil and skin and thereby help keep your complexion clearer and cleaner.

If you take that same piece of brown paper, rub it across your freshly wakened face, and discover barely a trace of oil, then you're a dry-skin type. This is not news to you, perhaps, but its implications bear directly on the increased sun exposure that naturally comes with summer living. In addition to stimulating the shed rate, sunshine also increases evaporation. Oily-skin types aren't troubled much by this, since their sebaceous oil, together with their moisturizers, naturally counter the sun's drying effects. Women with dry skin, however, can become even drier under the summer sun. Fortunately, summer humidity lessens the discomfort potential enormously. But the chance of pseudo-wrinkling, those fine, temporary wrinkles that stem purely from the unhindered evaporation of moisture from the skin, increases greatly in the summer sun. Your protection lies in the proper use of moisturizers (discussed below) plus prudently limited amounts of sun exposure.

Normal skin types don't experience too much change from season to season. Gauged by the brown paper bag, normal skin will leave a bit of oily residue, but not enough to turn the paper translucent. In fact, almost everybody has normal skin on at least some part of the face. It is common to have some dry areas, some oily ones, and still other regions that are simply normal. And each will require individual attention.

To sum up then, summer skin care, regardless of skin type, first means the increased attention to the need for PABA protection. And, for those with dry skin, it means extra moisturizing and particular caution, lest overexposure lead to undue dehydration.

What about summer makeup? This depends on a number of variables. If you use lots of makeup, the summer may well have no impact at all on your daily beauty regimen. Foundation makeup actually blocks out quite a lot of the sun's potentially damaging rays. Older women who've worn it all their lives always look more youthful than their counterparts who haven't. Surely the advent of summer is not reason in itself to change an elaborately evolved makeup regimen.

On the other hand, a summer tan does much of the job of a foundation makeup. And aesthetically, at least, it does it much better. Tans tend to clear the complexion (thanks to the aforementioned increase in the cellular shed rate) and provide a healthy, even color that can hide all sorts of minor imperfections. Many foundation makeups (including the one you should be using) contain PABA. If you're one of those women who do dispense with foundation makeup every summer, just be sure you aren't dispensing with the PABA protection at the same time. Remember, pure PABA dries invisibly and won't affect the appearance of your tan.

CORRECT CLEANSING

The season does not affect correct cleansing of the skin. Regardless of the time of year, and especially if you wear foundation makeup, you should be washing your face with soap and water. Nothing else can so effectively cleanse the skin of oil, pollution residues, old makeup, and dirt. So-called "cleansing creams" usually leave an oily residue that clogs the pores as much as whatever it was

pay. "Adequate protection" is something you have to determine by means of experimentation. If one product doesn't hold in the moisture well enough, then try one that's oilier.

A FEW WORDS ON THE WINTER SUN

Skiers and other winter sports enthusiasts must also be leery of the sun. Even though the winter rays are weaker, if they're reflected off a snowfield, they can still deliver a potent dose of ultraviolet tanning and burning rays. And wintertime air, not to mention the air in centrally-heated buildings, is about as humidity deficient as you can get.

Everything we've said about PABA protection in makeup applies equally under winter or summer skies. We don't believe winter cleansing regimens need be altered either. Moisturization, however, is doubly important in the winter because of the low humidity—and triply important if you plan to be out under a glaring and potentially dehydrating winter sun.

GOOD LOOKS FOR THE WARM WEATHER:
TIPS ON SUMMERTIME MAKEUP

What color? Think in terms of brightness and warmth when choosing summer makeup colors. The emerging tan will be adding its own glow, so you'll want to work with that, not against it. For a natural, sunny look you're also best advised to stick to monochromatic color schemes. Don't knock yourself out

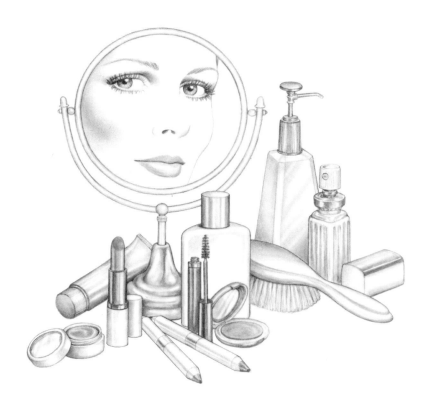

trying to exactly match your lipstick to your blusher, but do look for the same color family. And how do you pick your color family? As a general rule, for pale-skinned blondes pinky and mauve shades are most flattering; rose and terra cotta colors best suit dark redheads and brunettes; and darker brunettes look particularly well in reddish brown and bronze tones.

As noted earlier, many women get a good tan and then decide that foundation makeup is superfluous. By the beach or pool, this is usually the case, but indoors, unless both your tan and your skin tone are quite even, you may want to use that foundation anyway. If you do, make sure your summer foundation matches the color of your tanned face, or make it one shade darker. Alternately, you can substitute a bronzer for your foundation. Bronzers are available in stick or gel form and can do lots to even out and give added depth and resonance to your own natural tan. Whether you choose foundation or bronzer, always look for one with PABA among the listed ingredients. You may be calculating your effect in the indoors. But you'll still have to walk outdoors to get wherever you're going. Never forget that every single bit of sun exposure adds up in the course of a lifetime, and eventually it manifests itself in the form of cumulative sun damage to the skin.

Other elements of makeup must also be reevaluated in the context of summer sunshine and the general outdoors life of this time of the year. Blushers should be applied in those places where the sun would naturally strike the face —specifically, the tops of the cheeks and along the hairline. Don't dab the nose, unless you fancy looking sunburned. Eye shadow and lipstick, as mentioned earlier, will look best when they repeat, as closely as possible, the color of your blusher. Remember to search out PABA products as a matter of course. Lately we've seen lots of summer colors with names like cinnamon ginger and brick. These kinds of colors are definitely worth trying if they seem to suit your own natural coloration. (Blue and green eyeshadow are going to detract from a natural look.)

Lipstick is good for the lips at any time of the year. And since, as a natural sunblock, it protects admirably against sunburn and keeps the lips moist, you're well advised to wear it always in the sun, plus as a color complement to the rest of your summery makeup indoors or at night. Fortunately, PABA is contained in very many, if not most, good lipsticks.

How? How much? Now for some makeup tips. A handsome suntan can make daytime makeup exceedingly glamorous indeed. The first step is the application of either a bronzer or a foundation in a shade slightly darker than your winter choice. After application, set with translucent powder. Then hold a bright light overhead and observe where natural sheen occurs. Use highlighter at these points. Cheek hollows can be subtly shadowed with glowing bronze-toned blusher in cake form. Pick up the underbrow area with gold highlighter, and outline the lips with bronze pencil, then fill in with ruddy lipstick. Finish with a generous helping of lip gloss. Then curl your lashes with an eyelash curler and apply two coats of mascara. You can add a final theatrical touch by giving your eyebrows a bit of sheen with a touch of Vaseline.

For evening, you can intensify the effect of your summer makeup—and still not lose the natural look—by simply applying the color highlights with a slightly heavier hand. This will compensate for the tendency of artificial light to drain the appearance of color from the face—even from a nicely tanned

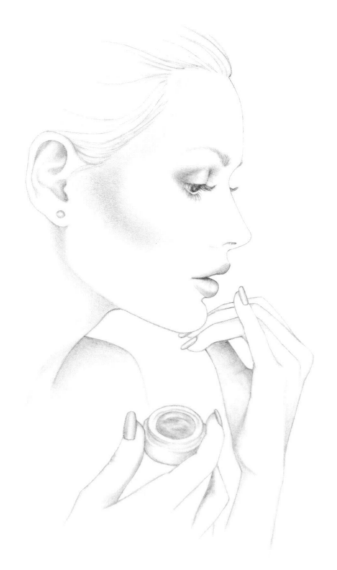

face. Gold highlighter is terrific for drawing attention to the same areas you normally reserve for your blusher, particularly the cheeks, hairline, and the region alongside the temples. Of course, you'll still use the blusher, but a subtle bit of added gold looks very exotic. Another trick, if you like a highlighter, is to put a little along the collarbone and on top of your shoulders. Eyeliner, by the way, doesn't always work so well with a tan. But lots of mascara always seems to be effective.

We wouldn't advise makeup at the beach, pool, tennis court, or wherever you expect to get lots of sun. Even though many makeups contain PABA, few contain enough to really protect you properly for the duration of a sunbath. And the opacity of certain blushers and highlighters can partially block tanning rays in such a manner as to leave you with a weirdly incomplete tan. Many products are advertised as waterproof. As far as mascara goes, this is doubtless a boon to swimmers who like glamorous eyes. But aside from mascara and lipstick (which is an excellent sunblock for sensitive lips that don't need a tan anyway), minimal makeup is called for whenever you're actively trying to get some color.

A last word on summer makeup: Since creamy formulations may change shape or consistency in the summer heat, it's always a good idea to buy products, where possible, in a powder form. As for the ones that only come in creams, you can at least try to keep them out of direct sunlight during the day, and maybe pop them into the refrigerator overnight.

SUNSHINE AND PERFUME

Two warnings come to mind immediately. The first refers to the phenomenon of photosensitization that we've mentioned before. In the case of perfume, there are often ingredients in the bottle that can give you an awful burn if you're sitting in the sun. Oil of bergamot, a common ingredient, especially in better quality perfumes, is perhaps the premier photosensitizer in the perfume trade. Therefore, in order to be on the safe side, *never* pat perfume all over yourself before a sunbath.

The second warning has to do with bugs. They love perfume. Especially bees and wasps, which you may find hovering all around you, looking for the pungent flower that you smell like. Even mosquitoes, flies, and sand fleas find perfumed women irresistible. So, bear this in mind.

The slightest climatic variations substantially change a perfume scent. In fact, heat and humidity play as large a part in determining how your perfume smells as does your own body chemistry. Warm, humid summer weather tends to make perfume sweeter and longer lasting—to bring out the base notes. This is why a spectacular scent that made heads turn in the cold weather may be altogether overpowering in the warm summer, or at a tropical resort. If your favorite perfume is running away with itself in this manner, try scenting lower pulse points instead of behind the ear. Heat, which disperses scent more freely, rises. Therefore try the back of the knees, thighs, and elbows and see what happens. Alternately, you can try the cologne or toilet water form of your favorite perfume. These contain the same perfume essence diluted with alcohol.

You might also try skipping direct perfume application altogether, and instead putting a few drops in your bath, maybe another drop in your moisturizer, another in your hand cream, etc. Of course, you won't want to do this and then go out into the sun, but it's a good way to achieve a subtle scent at night. You can also put the perfume onto the things you carry around with you. Hat brims, beach towels, even scented cotton balls tucked into a tote bag can have an excellent effect, being neither overpowering nor photosensitizing. Remember, however, that perfume smells differently on skin than on fabric. Give it a test before dowsing and dabbing everything and going off to the beach.

Finally, as with makeup, the sun can play havoc with perfume, even when it's in the bottle. So, keep your dressing table and everything on it in the shade throughout the day.

SHADES

Sunglasses are a must at the beach. While there are those who worry about looking like the reverse image of a raccoon, those threatened white circles around the eyes always seem to take care of themselves in the overall tanning process. And, of course, you don't wear them all the time anyway. Most optometrists believe going without glasses for limited periods of time in bright sunlight won't do any permanent damage. At the worst, it might cause such things as headaches, fatigue, and red or swollen eyes.

To be effective, sunglasses should filter out 85 to 90 percent of transmitted light. If you can see your eyes clearly reflected in a mirror while wearing your sunglasses, they are too light. Grey is considered the best color for maximum protection, with green and brown as second choices. Colors rated lowest on the protection scale are blue and purple. They transmit the color blue to your eyes, and blue is the closest shade to ultraviolet. Fashion colors, such as pink or orange, get low marks for glare protection, no matter how much they may flatter your eyes and skin. Besides, problems with color perception may result. Yellow gets mixed ratings; sports enthusiasts often select them for use on cloudy days to sharpen contrasts, but they don't do much to combat glare.

If you don't mind losing friends, you might consider mirrored sunglasses. They block out as much as 90 percent of the light, but many people loathe holding a conversation with someone while seeing only their own reflection throughout. Further, distortion can be a problem if you select the budget version, and the high-priced variety may be very high priced indeed.

More than $800 million is spent annually on sunglasses, most in the under $10 category. Meanwhile, designer glasses at $35 and up are capturing an ever-increasing share of the market. More than 80 percent of the glasses sold are plastic, which is lighter and more comfortable than glass. Glass, however, blocks those potentially dangerous ultraviolet rays far more effectively than plastic.

Determining color is just the first step in choosing a pair of sunglasses. Perhaps more important is lens type. Our favorite would have to be *polarized lenses*, in which two colored lenses are bonded in such a way as to cut both glare and reflected glare. They are heavier than the norm, but can be ground to prescription. *Photochromic glasses* are light sensitive and light responsive, which means they grow darker when exposed to sunlight, and grow lighter with decreasing light. Thus they are credited with preventing eye strain. While many experts rate them high for beach wear, they get low marks for driving because they change color at a relatively slow rate. Some take as long as 10 minutes to go from lightest to darkest. (Consider what that might mean coming out of a tunnel on a bright day.) Finally, there are *Ambermatic* sunglasses, which adjust to weather conditions. These lenses are brown when it's sunny and warm; dark silvery grey when it's sunny and cold, and amber when it's misty, to cut the haze and sharpen the outlines of whatever you're viewing.

Before you walk out of the store with any pair of sunglasses, be sure they are both distortion-free and comfortable. To test for distortion, tilt the lens to catch any straight line—an overhead fluorescent light fixture will do nicely—move them so the reflection runs across the lens, then look for any irregularities. If they pass that test, move on to comfort. If you wiggle your head, do they slide down? Do they press on the sides of your nose? Are they too loose or too tight at the temples? Is one side higher than the other? Are your cheekbones bearing most of the weight? Think of any pair of shoes you ever bought that seemed comfortable in the store and turned out to be agonizing after two hours of street wear, and do not leave the store until you are sure your sunglasses really fit.

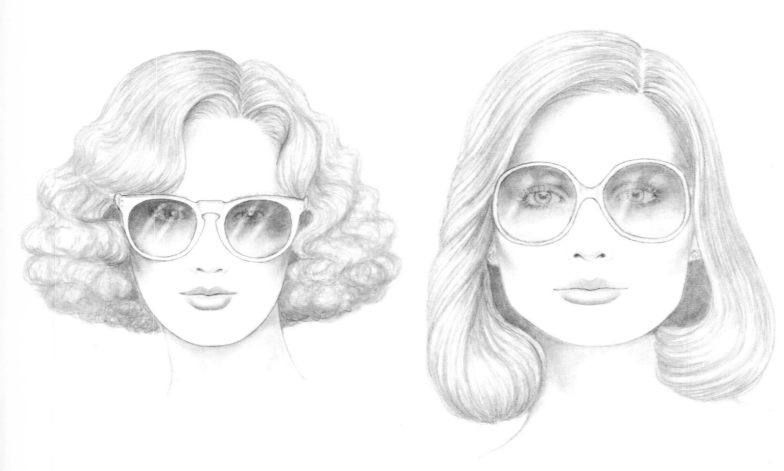

Then there's the shape of your shades to consider, and the aesthetic relation of that shape to the shape of your face. Women with oval faces are indeed blessed. Not only will just about any hairstyle look great, but they can also wear just about any shape of sunglass too. If there's one exception, it might bear on the thickness of the frames; skinny frames somehow don't look too good on an oval face.

If your face is square in shape, by all means shop for rounded sunglasses. Rounded shapes make a nice contrast with a squarish face, as do ovals and aviators. Angular-shaped glasses, however, will draw undesirable attention to the angularity of your face, and won't cast it in a flattering perspective.

Rounded faces, by contrast, carry off angular and squared sunglasses with great panache—the more geometric the glasses, the better.

And if your face is generally triangular or heart shaped, you're again advised to go for a style that compliments the shape of the face without overemphasizing it. Therefore, stick with aviators and ovals; square shapes are rarely flattering.

Having invested in a pair of possibly very expensive sunglasses, you should take pains to keep them scratch-free. You needn't worry about shattering, because there are government regulations about that. Given normal care, glasses won't split or crack either. Dropping them on a cement surface, however, or neglecting to store them in the case when you tuck them in your handbag can cause vision-impairing surface scratches. You should also wash your glasses regularly in soap and warm water, then dry them with a soft linen dish towel.

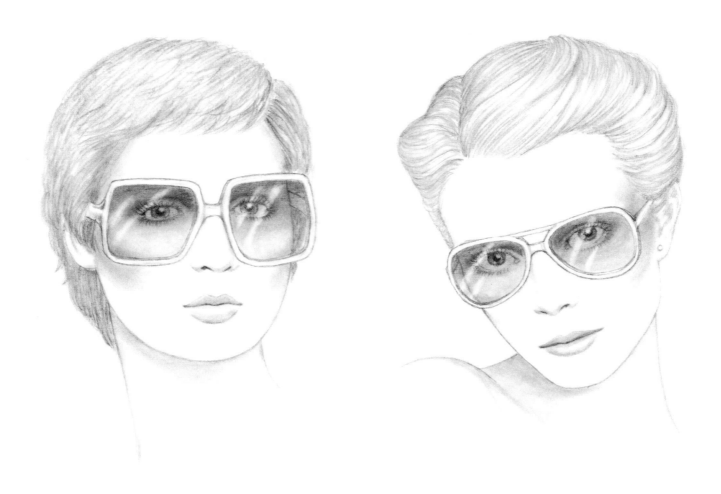

4. Sunny Beauty: Your Hair

The onset of sunny summer weather plunges many women into a positive frenzy of special seasonal hair care regimens. The point has been made by practically every stylist, colorist, and beauty magazine in the world that sun-exposed hair needs special care. Regrettably, the exact nature of this care is rarely explained in any coherent manner. Often the explanations are downright misleading.

Therefore, we're going to take a moment here to describe just how your hair shafts are constructed, just what makes them grow, precisely which elements of the summertime environment will affect them and which won't, and why.

HOW YOUR HAIR GROWS

Hair grows out of hair follicles, which are tiny organs buried deep in the dermis layer of the skin on your scalp. You have something on the order of 100,000 follicles on your head, and each one draws nutrients from the bloodstream, metabolizes them, and produces hair as a result. A hair shaft is rather like a fingernail in that its proper growth depends on a healthy generative organ (the follicle in the case of hair; the nail fold in the case of the nail), and in that both hair and nails are dead. Yes, your hair does *not* have a life of its own. A hair shaft is simply a lifeless protein structure comprised of several intricate layers.

You naturally possess several rather clever means of controlling and conditioning your own hair. The first is the structure of the shaft itself. In simple terms, each shaft consists of two somewhat soft inner layers (called the cortex and the medulla), which are wrapped with a protective outer layer called the cuticle. Hair cuticles under a microscope look like tiny coatings of incredibly intricate hinged shingles. When these little shingles lie flat, the hair looks

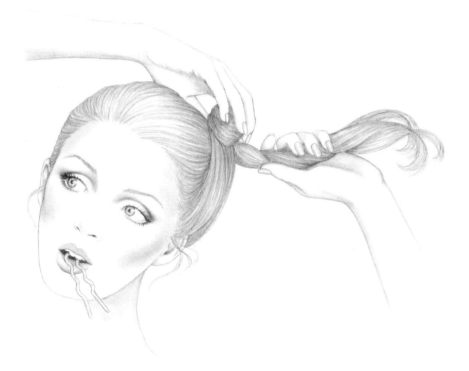

smooth, and glossy, is easy to run through with a comb or brush, and is generally manageable. When the shingles are opened, the hair looks dull, the shafts generate static electricity that makes them stand apart from one another, and the whole head of hair is tough to comb and murder to style. As long as your cuticles are kept closed and in good condition, however, they will naturally impart a smoothness and sheen to the hair.

You also have a built-in grooming system right on the top of your head. We refer to the oil glands whose openings are clustered around each hair follicle. Just as sebaceous oil glands help guard precious moisture elsewhere on the skin, so the oil glands on the scalp also prevent undesirable dehydration of the hair shafts. Hair is extremely porous and therefore quite sensitive to the changing moisture content of the air. If hair becomes unduly dehydrated by a dry environment, the result can be dull, unmanageable, even brittle hair. Scalp oil also lubricates cuticles and gives hair a natural sheen while also guarding against moisture loss.

Finally, a word about the color of your hair. The substance responsible for color is melanin, the same substance that determines skin color. Melanin in the hair, however, can't be stirred by ultraviolet light rays like it can in skin cells. This is simply because hair contains no living cells. The melanin is contained in the inner layers of the shaft, layers that are lifeless protein structures. The amount of melanin in the hair—and the color it presents to the naked eye—depends on the sort of follicles you inherited from your parents. Instead of being redistributed by the sun's rays, melanin in the hair can be oxidized away gradually. And this is why hair tends to lighten in the summer sun.

Having established these ground rules, let's take a look at the various environmental factors your hair is apt to encounter in sunny weather—with an eye to what you can and cannot do about each one.

THE SUMMER SUN

Hot summer sun beating down on your hair can bleach your hair color and dry out your individual hair shafts. These effects—and whether or not they're really serious—are obviously related to the amount of sun to which you expose your head. A certain amount of sun won't hurt you; perhaps you can even tolerate twice as much sun exposure as your best friend without any undesirable side effects. Sun tolerance, like hair quality, varies from individual to individual.

Many women count the sun's bleaching effects as a benefit. Sun-related melanin oxidation will not itself do any real damage to the hair. The hot infrared rays contained in the solar spectrum won't hurt you either—*unless* you bake yourself so much that you induce a condition of unmanageable dry hair due to dehydration. Even this can usually be countered easily with conditioners (a discussion which follows shortly).

If your hair is naturally dry and hard to manage, you should wear a scarf while you're sunning. In fact, you should make it a practice to shield your hair whenever it might be exposed to potentially dehydrating sunshine. If you have

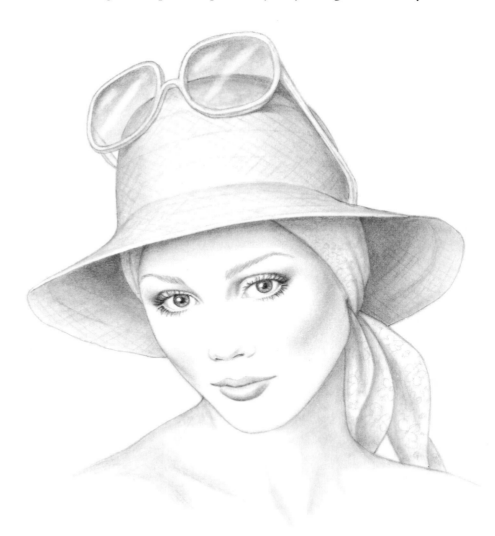

normal or oily hair, you needn't be so careful; you probably don't need to do much of anything about sunlight falling on your hair.

If you color your hair, then by all means take special pains to keep it out of the sunlight. Sunlight may bleach it or change it to some totally unexpected hue. The exact effect is a function of the type of dye you use, the type of hair you have, and the amount of sunlight to which you've been exposed. There are enough variables right there to preclude any accurate forecast and therefore to warrant extreme caution.

The texture and thickness of your hair are not critical factors in sun exposure because they don't bear much on either dehydration or bleaching.

SUMMERTIME HUMIDITY

Each one of your hair shafts will naturally react directly to humidity levels in the air around you. In the summertime, when it's often muggy, the moisture in the air will be sucked right up into each shaft. That's why moisture in the air makes curly hair fatter and frizzier, and artificially curled hair plumper and heavier, to the point that the curl falls out. By the same token, hair can easily become parched and brittle in arid desert environments or after a relentless session under the burning summer sun. Because it plumps up the hair shafts, humidity makes thin hair look a bit thicker. It has the same effect on thicker hair but the improvement in fullness isn't so noticeable. Usually what is most noticeable in humid weather is the difficulty you have trying to keep straight hair curly or flyaway hair under control.

POOL, LAKE, AND OCEAN WATER

Moisture is vital to the suppleness of hair. But swimming, ironically, usually dehydrates hair. This is because the process of evaporation that dries your hair after a swim also removes a bit of the moisture that was contained in each shaft before you took your dip. You might call this the "additional dehydration effect," and it is further exaggerated if the hair is allowed to dry directly in the hot sun. We are not saying that you shouldn't let your hair dry in the sun. But we are saying that repeated sun-drying will dry out the individual hair shafts. If you do it every day for weeks or months, your hair is going to have the consistency of hay.

The salt in seawater has a drying effect too—an effect that's exaggerated in combination with sunlight. And dried seawater can feel a little sticky in the hair. It's a good idea to rinse your head with fresh water on emerging from the ocean. If you aren't sunning by some posh beach cottage that comes equipped with a convenient cabana, then it's a good idea to bring a bottle of fresh water with you to the beach just for this purpose.

Like the salt in seawater, the chlorine in a swimming pool is also drying and will also increase the dehydration effect of sunshine on wet hair. Blondes must be particularly wary of chlorinated pools. Sometimes the chemicals can actually impart a greenish cast to blond hair, be it bleached or natural. This is an effect that is not always noticeable, and we understand that pool chemicals have been altered somewhat in recent years to avoid it. But the chance remains. So, if you're blond-headed, better wear a cap in the pool.

SUMMER BREEZES

Summer breezes sound so soft and cooling in the abstract, but the fact is that the good weather can mean a substantial increase in the amount of wind that blows through your hair. And wind—be it blowing through the open window of a car or off a romantic beach at sunset—will also contribute to the drying out of the hair through the process of evaporation. If you're having a problem with summer dryness, don't forget that those summer breezes can be part of the problem. So cover up against them.

PROTECTING YOUR HAIR FROM THE SUN

You need protection from two familiar factors: 1. sun, chemical, and wind-related dryness, and 2. solar-related melanin oxidation that can cause unwanted color changes.

The proper washing and drying of your hair won't alter much with the advent of sunny weather. All the ballyhoo about shampoos that are supposedly organic, exotic, pH balanced, or what have you is simply that—ballyhoo. All shampoo is basically soap, or a synthetic detergent that closely approximates soap. Just as soap cleans skin harmlessly and effectively, so soapy shampoos likewise clean the hair. There's nothing even in the cheapest shampoos that can hurt your hair. Although it really doesn't matter what shampoo you use, it does matter how many times you lather. Do it once, regardless of printed instructions to the contrary. A single lathering leaves intact between 60 and 80 percent of the natural oils on your scalp. A double lathering is unnecessarily drying.

Blow dryers are also unnecessarily drying. They have the dehydrating effect of pure sunshine magnified many times. Blow driers are very rough on the cuticles of your hair shafts—particularly the powerful ones, which can literally burn the cuticle away. When this happens, the inner layers of the shafts begin to unravel, resulting in unsightly split ends, unmanageability, and loss of sheen. Particularly in the summer, when your hair is probably exposed to more than its share of drying sunshine and pool chemicals, avoid a blow dryer whenever possible.

The real way to protect hair from most of the vicissitudes of summer sun exposure is through conscientious conditioning. Skin moisturizers seal moisture into the skin and protect it against evaporation, and hair conditioners act in much the same way. Most conditioners have an acid pH, which naturally closes down the cuticles and imparts a sheen to the hair. Conditioners also coat the individual hair shafts and protect them from moisture loss through evaporation.

Conditioners vary only slightly from creme rinses. These rinses are typically lighter solutions designed to be combed through freshly shampooed hair that's still damp. Creme rinses are great for smoothing cuticles, banishing tangles, and imparting shine and manageability. Conditioners do all this too, and they offer a greater measure of coating protection—especially conditioners with protein.

Use a conditioner immediately following every shampoo. In fact, it doesn't matter how often you shampoo, as long as you always protect yourself with conditioner. Some people are under the misapprehension that daily shampooing is connected to premature or increased hair loss. This is utter nonsense. Hair growth, together with its quality and its replacement rate, are determined by the genetically inherited strengths of your hair follicles. What's more, except for genetics the only things that affect follicles are those nutrients and hormones contained in your bloodstream. What you do on the surface of your scalp does not affect the way your follicles grow hair. So, if you have hair that needs daily washing, and you keep it well groomed with conditioners, you can rest assured that your frequent shampooings will not make your hair fall out.

Your own scalp oil, as mentioned earlier, is the body's natural hair conditioner. But the dehydrating elements of summer sun and water are more than many scalps can cope with. Therefore, you should not only follow every shampoo with a conditioning—the sort bottled for the shower are perfectly fine—but you may also want to give yourself a deep conditioning treatment every month. Again, if your hair isn't getting particularly dried out, or if you have abundant quantities of natural oil, this may not be necessary. But if you have dryness problems, use the deep conditioners. These products are available in drugstores everywhere. They usually involve the application of an oil of some sort (in truth, it doesn't much matter what kind of oil you use), kept on the hair for a given amount of time, often in conjunction with heat (which encourages absorption into the hair shafts).

All conditioners are designed to be rinsed out after application. And that means that in every case, much of the conditioning solution goes right down the drain. This is the major problem with that category of products known as shampoo-conditioners. Namely, their conditioning ingredients usually wash out along with the shampoo lather. Average drugstore conditioners leave adequate amounts of protection on your hair. Those with protein are best for all-around coating action, and they also give thin hair extra body. Those with oils—especially balsam—help naturally dry hair look shinier. Anybody can use protein conditioners, but people with thin or fine hair will find that oily or balsam conditioners make their hair unattractively lank. Remember that no conditioner will alter the nature or structure of your hair. All they do—to greater and lesser degrees—is protect the shafts from environmental factors by means of temporary coatings.

It may be, too, that your hair is either too dry, too fine, or has cuticles too damaged by chemical permanents, blow dryers, or coloring agents for it to sustain any sun exposure. In general, the more you've had done to your hair, the less able it is to withstand sun-induced dehydration. Even daily conditioning may not be enough. In that case, you'll simply have to wear scarves and hats in the sun and caps in the water lest the sunshine tip your delicate balance from processed hair to over-processed hair.

ADDITIONAL OBSERVATIONS ON SUMMER CUTTING AND LIGHTENING

The only cure for split ends is cutting them off. Once the cuticle starts to unravel, it cannot be permanently cemented back together. Of course, a certain amount of split ends is normal. Long hair, for instance, is oldest at the ends. The cuticles there have had the longest exposure to chemical and environmental drying. The coating action of conditioners, especially those containing protein, will minimize the appearance of split ends somewhat, but only until the next shampoo. And in the summertime, when exposure to sun and water is increased substantially, even the coating action of protein conditioners may not be enough.

You should be aware of this seasonal exacerbation of the year-round split end problem, and be sure to keep your hair properly trimmed during those months you expect the most sun exposure. You don't have to cut off a lot, just those ends that have started to unravel.

The summer sun may not help split ends much, but it's great for any hair lightening projects you may have in mind. Many summer blonding products are especially designed for use in the sun. You simply apply and sit outside as usual. The resultant blonding is many times more effective than that achieved by simply sitting in the sun. If the hair is properly conditioned during the period these products are used, it will not be any the worse for wear.

The sunny season is a good time to have your hair professionally streaked or lightened, too. Natural sunlight just helps the salon effect along. The sunny season is not, however, the time to have your hair permanented. Again, the effect of the heat and oxidizing rays is hard to calculate, and permanent waving constitutes a fairly significant assault on the structure of each hair shaft. Excessive sun exposure following such treatments will inevitably lead to unwelcome problems of dryness, if not to a partial reversal of the wave itself.

SUNSHINE AND HAIRSTYLES

Since the sun is hot, there's lots to be said for short haircuts. But since the hot weather can also mean lots of swimming, there's even more to be said for easy haircuts. Styles that can be simply imposed on hair still damp from the pool are not only convenient but also have a spiritual kinship with the whole idea of summer and outdoorsiness.

Brushes are tough on wet hair. It does not matter if the bristles are natural or nylon. The problem lies with the profusion of bristles and their frequent sharpness. Too much brushing with bristles that are too dense or too sharp can yank hair right out of the scalp. Or, it can fracture the cuticles and encourage split ends. The best way to style the hair—especially when it's wet—is with a comb whose teeth are widely spaced and blunt. If you've followed our advice and assiduously used your conditioner or creme rinse, there should not be any problems with tangles.

What follows now is a baker's dozen of summer hair styles for various hair lengths. Each style is illustrated and accompanied with a few words of instruction. While the style that suits you best will depend on the length, texture, and condition of your hair, they're all well suited to summer living, and most can be worn either wet or dry. Each is accompanied with a few words of instruction. Enjoy.

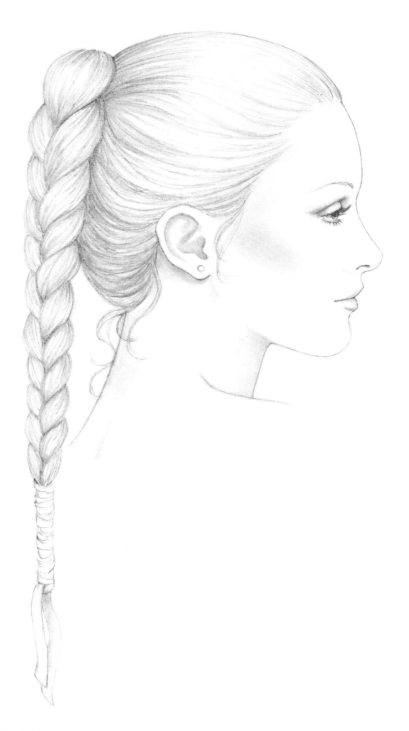

The thick braid. This one's easy to do straight from the shower, fresh from the pool, or with hair that's already dry. Simply bend over, gather your hair at the crown, and plait it into a single fat braid. As it narrows at the bottom, you can wrap it with any number of things—ribbon, colored string, beads, thread, whatever—and tie the wrappings at the bottom.

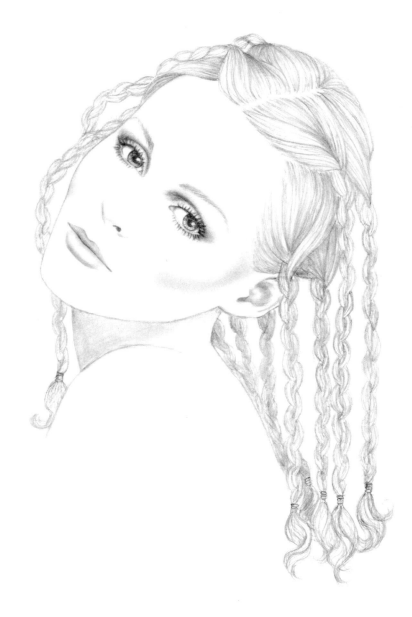

Multiple braids. This one's cute, but a little time consuming, and not every-one can carry off this sort of thing. The bonus of the style is that if you braid your hair while it's wet, you'll get a headful of curls after your braids have out-lived their usefulness. Your first step is to part the hair in the middle and address yourself separately to each side of the head. Basically, you're going to make three (possibly four) additional parts down each side of the head. Each part will be parallel to the initial part at the crown. Make your first one below the crown, and separate the hair into six equal strands. Pin three of them aside while you braid the other three; then take the pinned strands and braid them. You now have two braids, which should be pinnned up and out of the way so that you can work on the next layer. Again, you'll make a part parallel to the last one and lower down on the head. Separate the hair, and pin and braid as

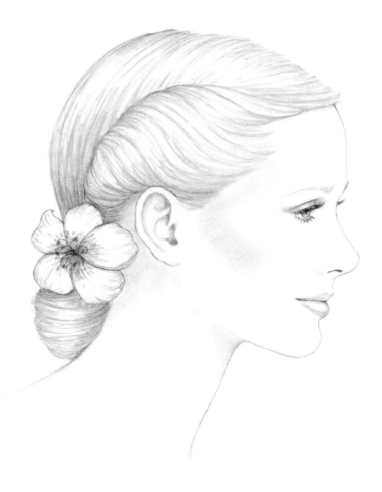

above. If you have lots and lots of hair, you may have to repeat this sequence more than three times on each side of the head. For most women, however, three layers should do it. Number and sequence is not so important, but neat sectioning gives more of a stylish look.

The chignon. If not done with wet hair, this one may require a setting lotion. Comb the hair smoothly back, twisting each side into a coil, reinforcing the coil with pins where needed. Secure at the back with a coated elastic band and hairpins. Then roll up the extra hair at the back of the neck and secure with pins as well. Garnish the roll at the neck with a flower, real or fake—it won't matter a bit.

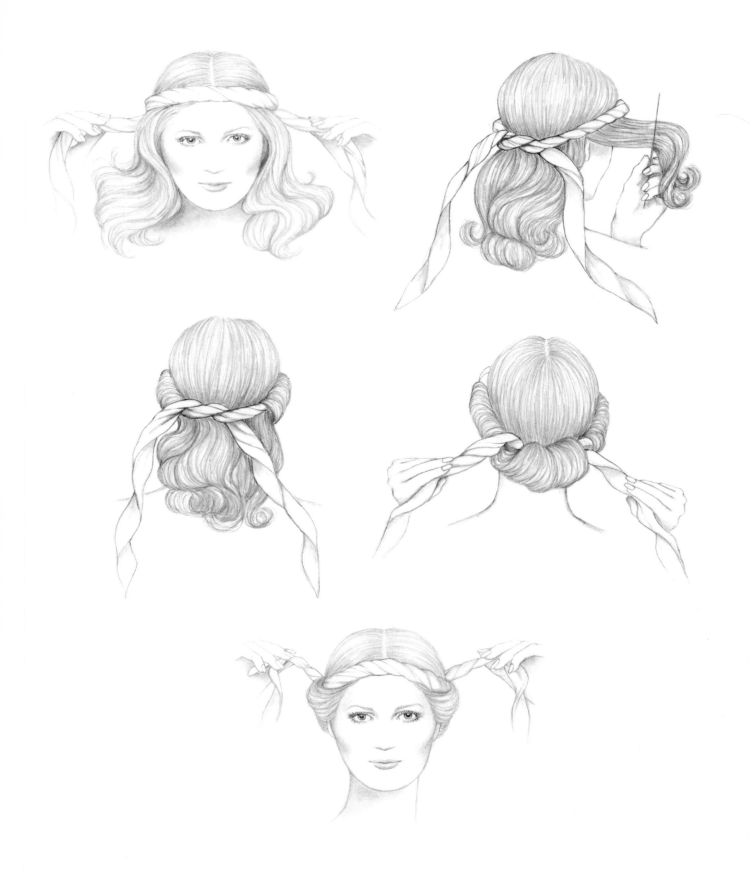

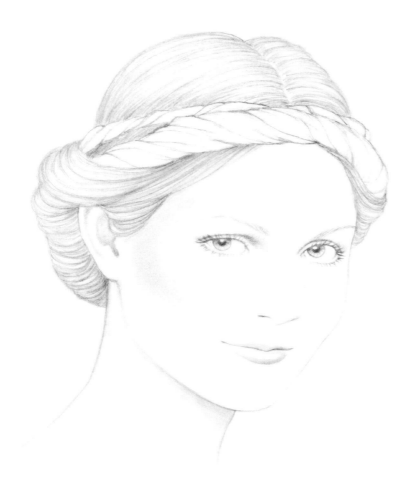

Scarf-rolled hair. Here's an idea that's terribly summery—and you're not likely to run across another woman in the same room who knows the secret. First, part your hair in the middle and comb it straight down either side of your head. Next, take a large cotton scarf and twist it into a rope. Holding the scarf at either end, center it at or near the hairline in front, and loop the ends in back. Then take a wide section of hair at one side of the front, comb it into a manageable section, and tuck it over and through the scarf. Do the same with an equivalent strand on the other side. Then place a mirror behind you, and, alternating sides evenly, tuck the remaining hair over and through the scarf in the same manner. You'll probably need a comb to neaten the ends as you progress. When all the hair has been neatly rolled around the scarf, pull the two ends back around to the front, knot them, and tuck them down under the front portion above the forehead.

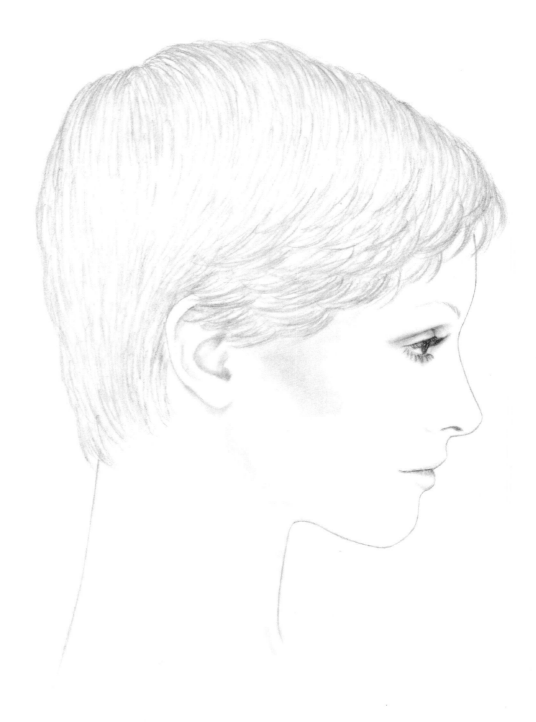

The layered cap cut. A short cut that's both stylish and easy, because it all lies in the cut. Trimming is obligatory every five or six weeks, but with hair like this, you won't be wasting much time wondering how to arrange it. Simply comb or brush it into place, wet or dry.

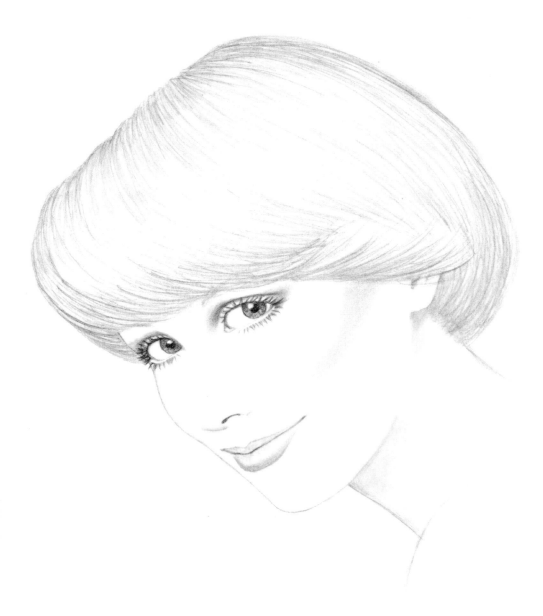

The bowl cut. Not quite as carefree as it looks, though a great style if your hair has lots of native body. It will probably require a bit of additional fussing with a blow dryer and comb. If you don't think your hair will dry naturally to a fullness like this, then it's probably better to shop for another style. Daily blow drying is definitely *not* what you want to do to summer hair that's getting lots of sun exposure.

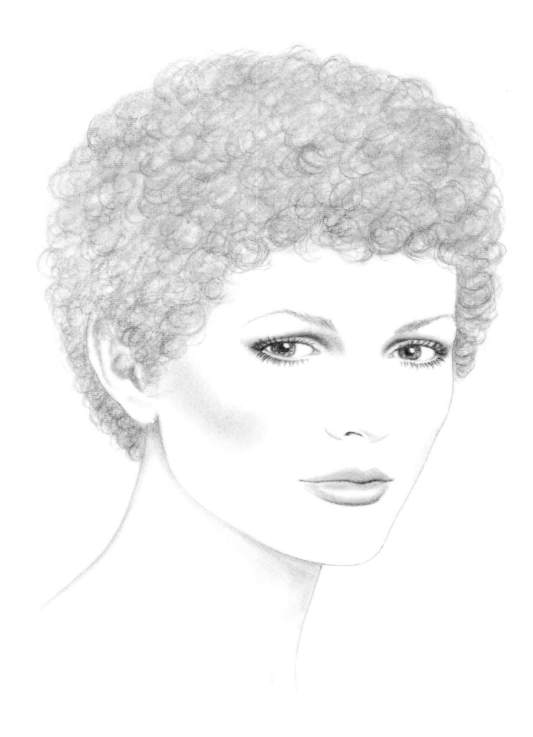

Curly and natural. Thank God it's finally fashionable. If you have lots and lots of natural curls, relax and enjoy them, and be the envy of your friends. Again, the secret is a good cut, kept fairly short. Arrange it with a wide comb before it dries, or fluff with the fingers.

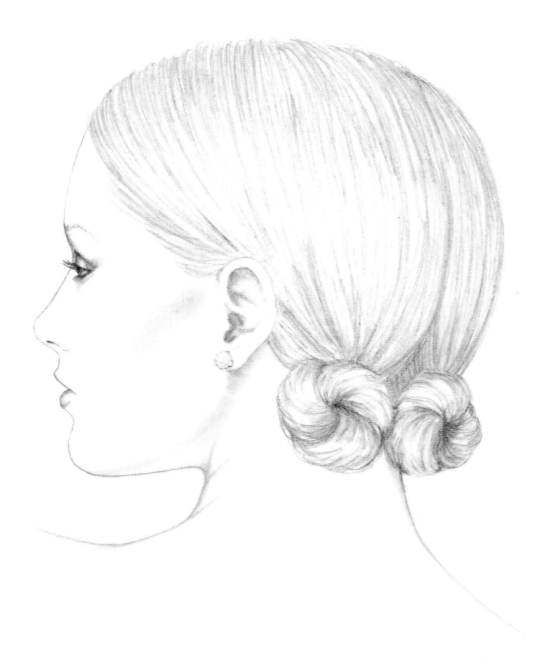

The double chignon. Simply a variation on the chignon described above, this style is good if you have a little more hair. Part the hair in the middle, comb it all slickly back on both sides, make two buns and pin them up side by side.

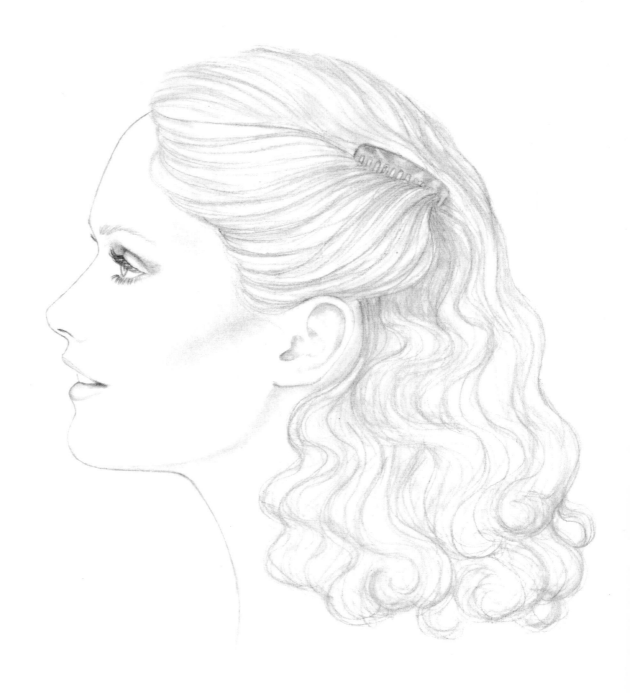

Something for hair that's long and very curly. Just comb it back from the forehead and hold it softly in place with combs (the more decorative the better) placed on the sides of the head. Even if your hair is straight, you can achieve the same effect by braiding it during the day and releasing it at night.

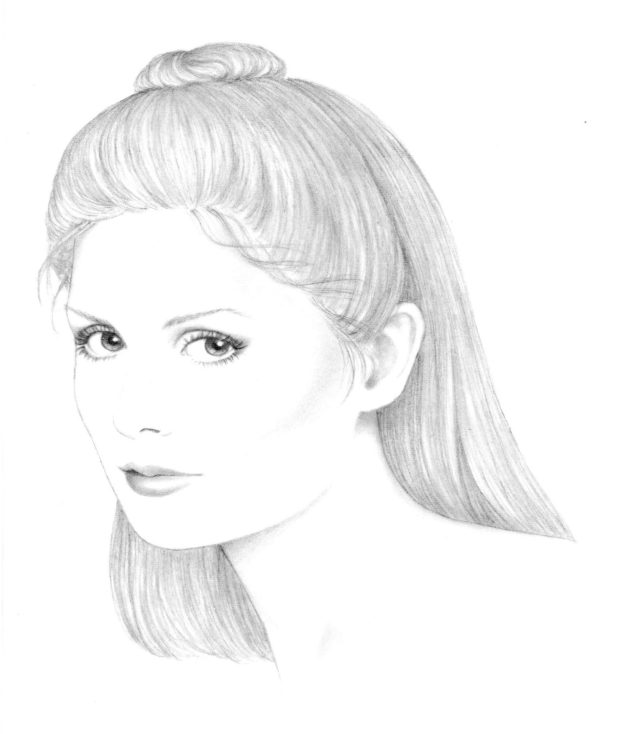

Something for hair that's long, straight, and heavy. Gather a large section of hair from the top of the head loosely at the crown, twist it into a small casual curl, and pin it down off center. Then just let the rest fall smoothly down your back. This is a great way to show off luxuriant shining hair.

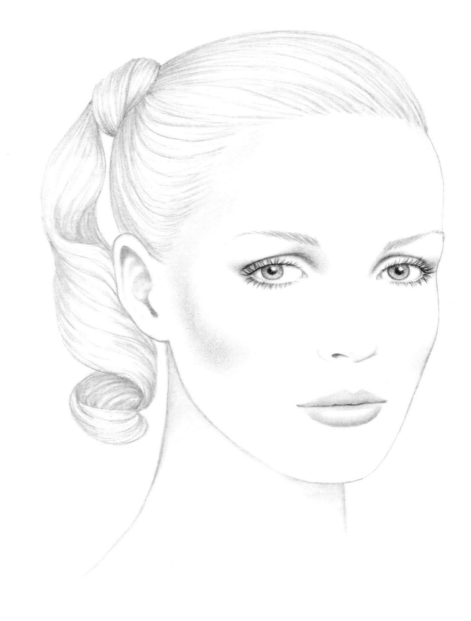

The pony tail. It's not old hat if you pull it off to one side, curl it into a loose twist at the base, and cover up the elastic with a little swag of hair. This can even look rakish, and more so if you put one on each side, or two on one side!

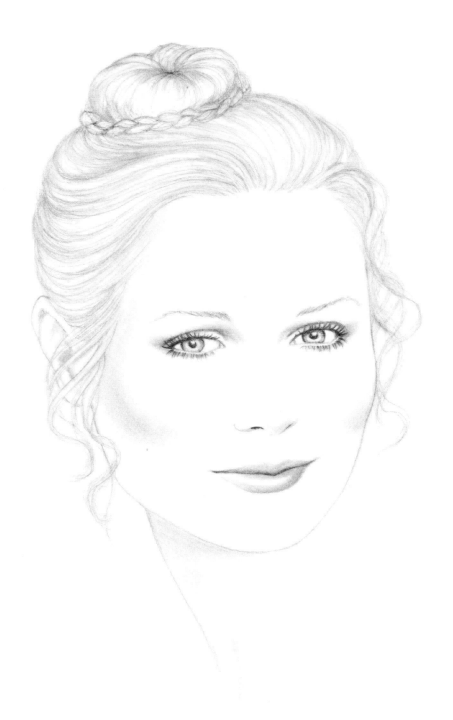

Upstairs/downstairs. What with Edwardian elegance back in style, this sort of old-fashioned look can be just the ticket. All the hair is combed back from the forehead, then gathered up completely onto the top of the head in a circular topknot (optionally encircled with a braid). Little tendrils along the side are actually encouraged to escape so as to soften the effect.

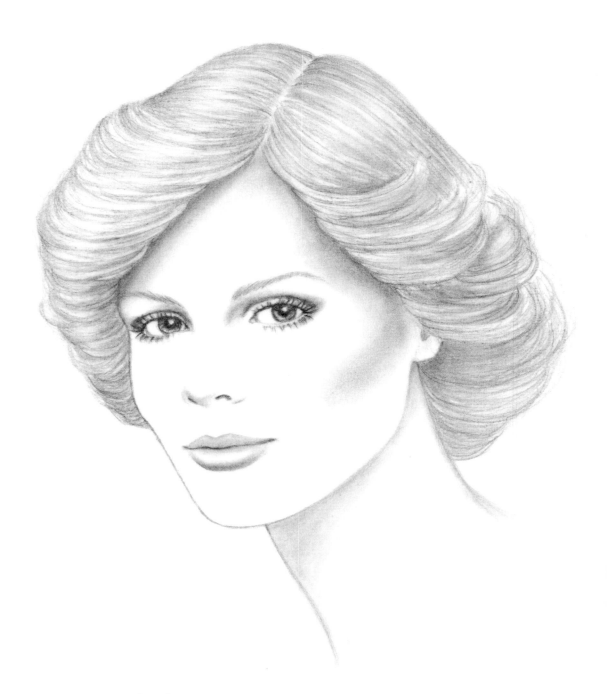

Blow dryer fullness. Fun, but only for special evenings. That's because regular use of blow dryers is entirely too drying for the hair at any season of the year, and especially during the sunny season. Still and all, this brushed-back look of fullness—easily accomplished either by training the blower on your comb or by using a special styling attachment that comes on many new blowers —not only looks glamorous, but is fairly fast work to boot. If your hair has sufficient body, and if it's quite short, you can probably achieve the same effect by brushing it with a little setting lotion applied while the hair is damp.

5. Sunny Beauty: Your Body

Shed those heavy winter clothes, put on your bathing suit, and stand before a full-length mirror. There now, that should be motivation enough to get to work on that body! Fortunately, sunny summery weather is the perfect time to color up pale winter complexions, to moisturize dry winter skin, to manicure rough winter feet, and to otherwise render yourself irresistible.

SUMMERTIME PRESCRIPTION #1: THE BEAUTIFYING BATH

Warm weather humidity does lots by itself to counter the typical dry skin problems—rough spots, flaking, discomfort—that afflict nearly all of us during the winter. But hot, dehydrating infrared rays from the summer sun can bake away more surface skin moisture than humidity levels alone can provide. Of course, if you spend the whole summer in the shade, you won't have a dryness problem. But what fun would that be? Especially when the key to summertime skin protection (and beautification) is as simple as turning on the water in the tub.

Well, actually, there's a little more to it than that. There's a right way to bathe and a wrong way. And what you do during the first five minutes following your bath has a critical effect on its success in protecting summer skin. Baths, in terms of thorough moisturization, are better than showers, but if you don't have a good tub you can still apply most of our advice to a shower.

The Edwardians and the Victorians had the right idea when it came to bathtubs. They made them big and deep. In more recent times, tubs have become scandalously shallow and short—entirely too much so for our purpose.

Since moisturization is firstly a matter of soaking yourself in water, you want a big tub into which you can fit all of yourself.

Summer bath water must not be too hot. It is an unpleasant fact that too hot, too long baths actually lead to dehydration. This is because hot water opens the pores, and open pores allow moisture to begin rapidly evaporating out of the skin the minute you step from your bath. Prune fingers are a commonplace symptom of bathwater dehydration. Especially in the summer, your bathwater should be lukewarm, maybe even slightly tepid. You'll also have to limit your time in the tub. Ten minutes is about the outside limit for any hot-weather bath, especially if you've been sunning during the day.

Speaking of sun exposure, schedule your bath for that time of day immediately following your stint at the beach, by the pool, on the courts, or on the fairway. This way you'll be replacing lost moisture when it's most needed. In fact, the sooner you can get into your tub the better. The really unwanted evaporation starts in earnest as soon as your perspiration dries.

Bathwater additives—beads, gels, bubble baths, scents, etc.—are usually nothing more than oily additives. As such, they will help seal moisture into the skin, which is precisely what any sort of moisturizer does. The trouble with bathwater additives is that putting them into the tub before you get in will actually inhibit the penetration of moisture into your thirsty skin. This is because oily water won't sink in so well. Our advice is to draw the tub at a desirably low temperature, get in, soak for a few minutes, and *then* add the

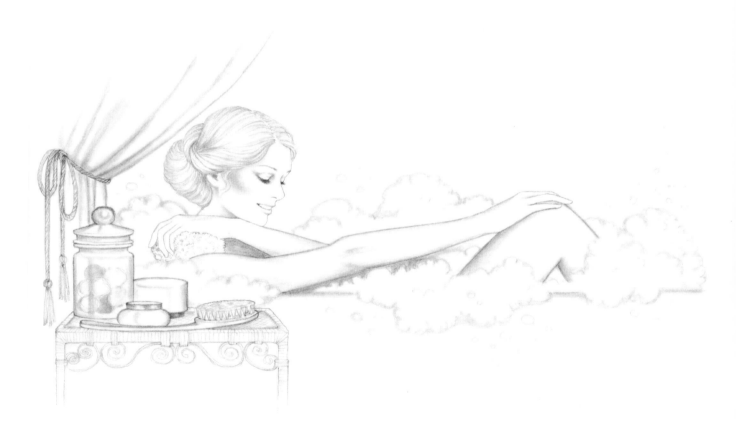

bath oil, bead, gel, or whatever. As the additive dissolves, it can impart its moisture-protective oiliness to the bathwater, and leave an evaporation-resistant residue clinging to your skin even after you're out of the tub and dry.

What about soap? To be sure, soap cuts through oil (natural as well as added) and is indeed drying to the skin. However, you're not going to get clean without it. Our advice is to choose a soap containing oil or cream (it doesn't matter which type) or one with a superfatted formula designed specifically for dry skin. Use your soap sparingly, and put it aside in the dish before you pour your bathwater additive into the tub. The oil in the additive will help counter the natural, if necessary, degreasing effect of the soap.

Stepping from a bath like this leaves the body clean, the skin nicely hydrated, and the soul soothed. But now comes the really important part. The minute you're out of the tub, pat yourself lightly dry with a soft terrycloth towel (a little residual surface dampness is okay). Then take your favorite moisturizer and apply it immediately. In fact, there are more moisturizing products on the market than any nation needs. Hand lotions are really not too different from body lotions, which, in turn, don't differ much from facial moisturizers. All these products merely attempt (with varying degrees of success) to erect a semi-impervious barrier between your hydrated skin and the dehydrating air that surrounds it. The sooner you apply your after-bath moisturizer, the less chance the air will have to evaporate moisture from your skin. Be sure to do your whole body, not just those areas of traditional dryness (elbows, knees, hands, and the like). Really massage yourself well. Daily baths followed by daily total moisturization of this sort will do wonders to promote smooth and supple summer skin.

What if your tub is pathetically shallow or you're just a shower person? Well, follow our advice on lowering water temperature, limiting time in the water, using a not terribly drying soap and not too much of it. Apply your moisturizer within minutes of turning off the water, and you'll achieve essentially the same good results. The real key is getting that moisturizer onto your still slightly damp skin—and getting it on fast. Followed daily, a bathing regimen like this will keep skin smooth and conditioned, and protect it from the dehydrating heat of the summer sun.

HAIR REMOVAL

Bathing suits, halter tops, the frequent absence of pantyhose, etc., make summertime hair removal a matter requiring particularly close attention. Unless and until currently held images of beauty change significantly, this situation isn't likely to alter much either. The fact is, really sexy female bodies are, by definition, smooth and hairless. The pubis and the head are the *only* exceptions.

Some women are lucky. They have hardly any body hair. Others aren't so lucky, and for them, hair removal is a chore that simply cannot be neglected. Herewith, the six major methods of hair removal.

1. *Shaving.* It is an old wives' tale that shaving causes hair to grow back faster and/or darker. The rate and nature of hair growth depends on the genetically determined character of hair follicles, plus the presence of various hormones and nutrients in the bloodstream. It really has nothing to do with shaving.

Besides, shaving happens to be the cheapest, fastest, and easiest way to groom those parts of the body that require regular hair removal. Make it a part of every bath or shower. It's simply not that time consuming. Worried about occasional nicks or cuts? Simply go to a drugstore and get yourself a styptic pencil. These cheap and effective little items use aluminum salts to instantaneously stanch the flow of blood from nearly every sort of minor shaving cut. Men use them all the time, and there's no reason you shouldn't, too.

Shaving is, however, abrasive. It won't be comfortable on skin you've allowed to burn. Shaving is also traditionally followed by alcohol-based aftershave preparations. These are extremely drying and are to be avoided at all costs. Simply rinse the shaved area well, and moisturize as you would the rest of your body.

When is the best time to shave? While you're *in* your bath or shower. Is there any particular type of shaver to use or avoid? Twin-bladed systems are too abrasive even for heavily whiskered male faces. For you, they're that much worse. Stick to single blades, and keep them sharp. Disposable razors are cheap and usually have long handles that are particularly easy to use. Which areas of the body are most efficiently smoothed by means of shaving? Legs, thighs, underarms, and lower abdomen. But can other parts of the body be safely shaved as well? Yes, unless your technique is so heavy handed that you irritate delicate skin. (*Note:* While electric razors are fine for a quick touch-up, they don't usually give a very close shave. Also, they're certainly to be avoided in the bathtub!)

2. *Bleaching.* This doesn't remove hair, of course. But for all intents and purposes, bleached hair might just as well not be there, because it's virtually invisible. You can get good, inexpensive bleaching kits at any drugstore. Bleach preparations are ideal for facial and arm hair. Use these kits regularly, but never immediately prior to extended sun exposure. They employ strong chemicals—especially hydrogen peroxide—whose effect in combination with sunlight is difficult to predict.

3. *Waxing.* There are hot wax kits you can cook up and apply at home, and there are waxing strips designed for home use, too. But you'll undoubtedly get a far superior job by going to a beauty salon. Some establishments even specialize in waxing, often in combination with electrolysis.

For those who don't know already, the process involves application of molten wax to the area where hair is to be removed. The wax cools, hardens, and is then ripped from the skin, taking the hairs with it. Not excruciating, to be sure, but also not very pleasant—especially in the case of bikini waxing, wherein certain tender areas are treated so that revealing bikinis may be prevented from revealing anything other than smooth skin. It must also be noted that hair removal by means of waxing is in no way permanent. The hairs are yanked out by the roots alright, but the follicle that grew them is very much intact down there in the dermis layer of the skin. It's just a matter of time—typically a few weeks—until new hairs emerge again on the surface.

4. *Depilatories.* These products employ another strong chemical, this one called thioglycolate. This substance has the ability to actually dissolve hair. Interesting to note, thioglycolate is also employed in permanent hair dyes. It effectively opens the outer layers of the hairs, thereby allowing dye chemicals to enter. Hair dyes, however, have neutralizers to arrest the action of thioglycolate. Depilatories require no such neutralizing action. They are simply allowed

to soften the hairs to a point where they can be wiped right off the surface of the skin.

Depilatories are safe for most people, although there are naturally some (although not many) who will have allergic reactions. Don't use depilatories in the sun, or immediately prior to sun exposure. Again, it's just too hard to predict whether or not they'll react adversely in the presence of prolonged direct sunlight.

Some people feel that depilatories slow the growth of body hair. Strictly speaking, this isn't so. However, the top of a shaved hair is at a level practically equal to the surface of the skin. Hairs removed with depilatories are dissolved right down to the buried follicle itself. Thus, new growth must travel a bit of subsurface distance before emerging atop the skin. Result: There is a small additional time delay before obvious reappearance of the hair when depilatories are used.

Depilatories are recommended for legs, and that's about all. Using them is a little sloppy and time consuming, too. If you really want our opinion, we'd say stick with a razor instead.

5. *Electrolysis.* This treatment has traditionally been the province of the professional beauty operator. Nowadays, however, you can do it at home, too. Electrolysis represents an approach to unwanted hair different from any we've discussed so far. It is a method wherein a tiny platinum needle is inserted directly into the hair follicle (yes—ouch!), a tiny electrical current is released, and the follicle is usually fried to death. Is that really the case? Will it never again grow a hair? Well, yes and no. *The generally accepted rate of regrowth is 40 to 60 percent!* In other words, electrolysis may kill about half the follicles treated.

Besides the discomfort, it's expensive. And the regrowth factor requires return visits over extended periods of time. However, when all is said and done, it really does work. And this is proven by the legions of women who annually employ this method to rid themselves of unwanted hair.

Is electrolysis the answer to permanent hair removal everywhere on the body? On the face, probably yes. Elsewhere, it depends. Large skin areas with fairly widespread hair growth are not good candidates for electrolysis treatment. It's painstaking work, costly, and too slow going for legs, arms, or certain thighs.

You can do your own electrolysis at home by means of a battery-operated needle arrangement that allows you to penetrate your own follicles, fry them, pluck out the hair and hope for the best. There are several home electrolysis tools on the market: This is the type of item you find advertised in the mail order section of women's magazines.

Still another alternative to professional electrolysis is professional treatment in which ultra-sonic waves are substituted for the electric shock. Again, the follicles must be invaded one at a time by a tiny needle, but some people claim that this technique is considerably less painful. Just how much will vary from one individual to another.

6. *Tweezing.* By now there's probably nothing about tweezing that you can't infer from the data above. It yanks hairs out without really affecting the follicles that grow them. It's obviously ill-suited for extensive areas, but will work well for spot removal. Tweezing is also the safest, simplest, and most manageable way to remove hairs from the brows.

SUMMERTIME FEET

Summer means more of you is on display, including your feet. They may have been out of sight (in shoes and stockings) and out of mind all winter long, but now you have to take care of them—careful care, too. Most men find lumpy callused feet with weird toenails to be a definite turnoff. No matter—conscientious pedicuring can be fun. It contributes to a feeling of being pampered, even if it's you doing your own pampering instead of some sexy man servant with oiled muscles and a turban.

A proper pedicure is obtainable in many beauty parlors, but you can easily do it yourself. Be sure to do it right. That means doing it once every 10 days or 2 weeks. Allow 45 minutes for the process, the first 20 of which to be spent soaking the feet in warm, soapy water. This softens the skin and makes calluses easier to tackle. Here now is a 7-point checklist, with illustrations, to enable you to keep your feet looking as good as possible.

1. Correctly soak and soften. Brushing callused areas encourages water absorption.

2. Carefully push back softened cuticles with an orange stick. Wrapping the tip in cotton is optional; some women find it more comfortable. The point of this is to give the nails a tidier look, *not* to scrape away, clip off, gouge out, or otherwise obliterate the cuticle itself.

3. Rub calluses with a pumice stone. Keep your soapy water for this, as it makes the rubbing easier. In truth, callus removal by means of home pumice treatments is a process that requires a number of pedicures to complete. Once it's complete though, you'll have to keep the callused areas constantly maintained.

4. Now, clip your nails. Use a special toenail clipper, and make the cuts straight across. Cutting the sides down risks infecting the delicate tissue that butts up against the sides of the nails.

5. Buff each nail with a nail buffer. Then just leave them that way, or,

6. Paint them with the same color you use on your fingernails. If you polish your toenails, you'll find the process is made somewhat simpler by separating the individual toes with cotton balls, with a twist of tissue (as illustrated) woven between the toes.

7. Once the polish has completely dried, massage the feet with moisturizer. Actually, the threat of dry skin on the feet shouldn't worry you too much. But moisturizers smell good, feel nice, and do hold in a certain amount of moisture that can make the skin more supple. All of which are certainly good reasons to use one—any one—on your feet.

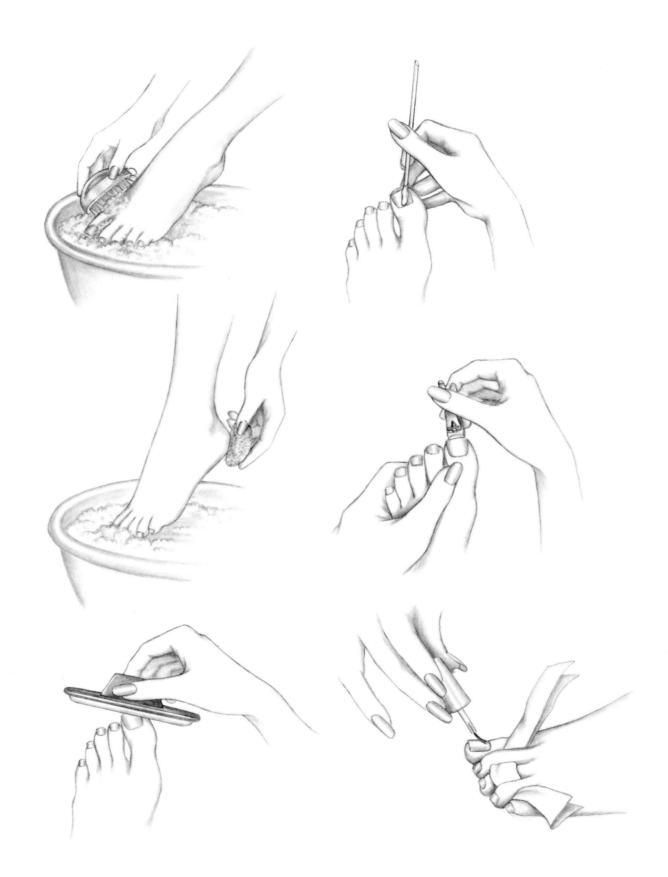

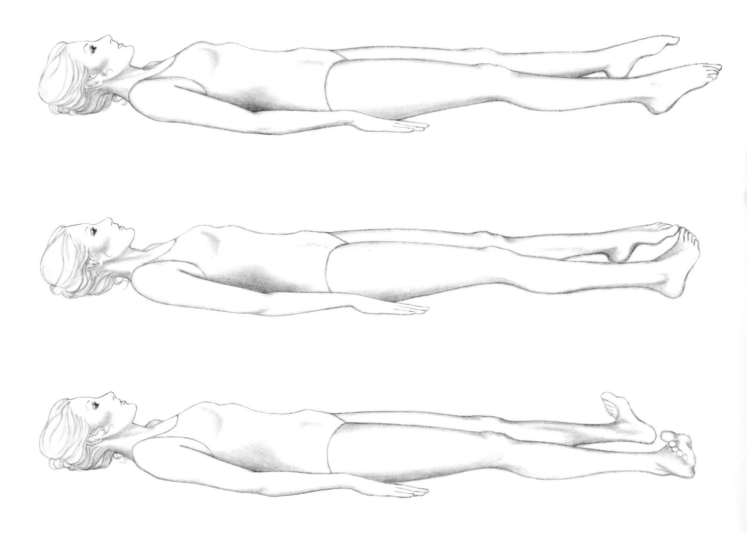

After your pedicure, you might like to try a few foot stimulation exercises. They're fun and feel wonderfully good on well-pedicured feet.

1. Lie down flat, and point your toes straight ahead in line with your body. Hold them for a moment, then touch your big toes together, then pull both feet up and out so as to point your heels straight down. Hold that for a moment and repeat the whole thing. Recommended dosage: twelve complete toe and heel points.

2. Sit in a chair and extend your legs straight in front of you. Rotate both feet clockwise simultaneously. After twelve full rotations, rotate them both counter-clockwise.

3. Stand on top of a telephone book, toes extending over the edge. Use those toes to try and grasp the edge of the book. A few tight grasps is all that's needed.

4. Walking barefoot on the beach is one of the best possible exercises for feet used to being confined in shoes most of the year. The sand not only feels

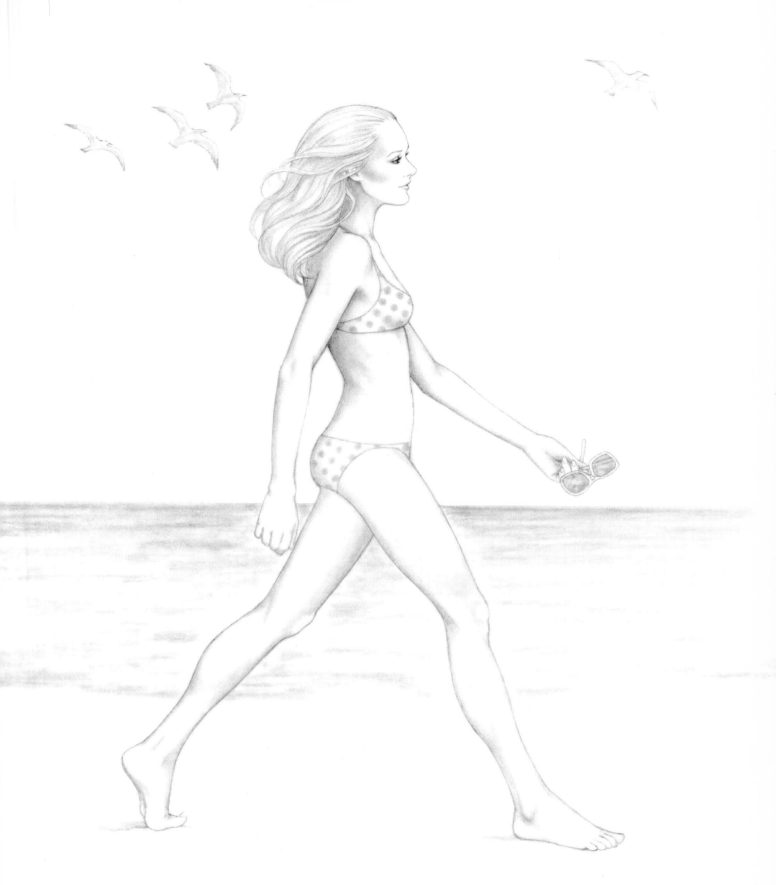

great, it gives all your foot muscles a workout. The best sand is soft sand. And since soft sand is usually well above the wave line, take your beach walk before the sun has a chance to make that sand uncomfortably hot.

Before we leave the subject of summer feet, a few further observations are in order. The first concerns the occasional discomfort some people experience after going barefoot for a while. The cause of this is high-heeled shoes, which, by elevating the heel, have shortened the tendon muscles of countless women and men. The effect varies from one calf to another, but almost without exception, people who have grown up in societies where shoes are worn will experience some discomfort (albeit often barely noticeable) if they go without them for a spell. This applies to men, too. Witness the obligatory built-up heel in running shoes. Male runners may not wear heels as high as women's during regular activities, but their everyday shoes still have heels that are high enough to require a build-up in the running shoe. And as every runner knows, he or she who runs in an un-built-up tennis shoe gets painful tendonitis. Simply because the foot is unaccustomed to the extra stretching that comes with heelless shoes. Walking around barefoot can result in the same phenomenon, an uncomfortably stretched tendon.

Some final advice: Many people are tempted to go sockless in the summer. As long as your shoes have cotton or canvas tops, this is fine. But leather shoes, or fashions that fully enclose the foot, are too hot and too potentially abrasive. Wear pantyhose or peds or anklets. And don't think you can just sprinkle powder in closed shoes and be comfortable. After a few weeks of that, the insides of your shoes will develop a most unappetizing paste.

RANDOM THOUGHTS ON SUMMER CLOTHES AND JEWELRY

You'll be happier in hot weather if your clothing is cool. Light colors, since they reflect the rays of the sun, will deflect considerably more solar heat than darker colors. Natural fibers are cooling, too, since their woven structure breathes better than synthetics. (And then there is the problem of the tenacity with which some polyesters cling to old odors.)

Loose fits are good for summer, too; the idea being that the more air movement between your clothes and your body, the cooler you'll be. Exotic caftans and burnooses not only look arresting, they're singularly well-suited to scorching weather.

As for jewelry, less is definitely more when it comes to sitting out in the sun. Gold or metal jewelry not only looks oddly heavy without lots of clothing, but it gets dangerously hot. An exception is the fine gold chain, which is too thin to get hot. These chains can look particularly sexy when worn around the waist with a bikini.

White looks great against tanned skin, especially by romantic evening light. Summer, by its very nature, is a relaxing time, and that means you can relax your notions of good jewelry a bit, too. All sorts of things work in the context of a sun-drenched weekend house or vacation resort. Even if you're normally conservative with your jewelry, the sunny season is the time to try things like cork, shells, colored strings and cords, chunks of lucite, in short, anything that catches your fancy.

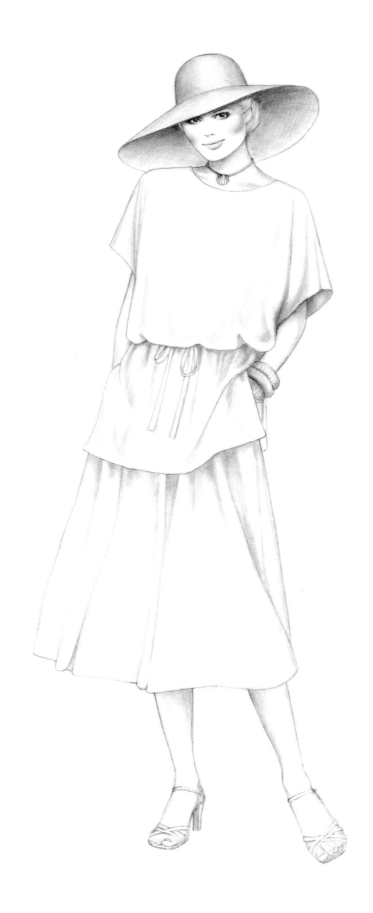

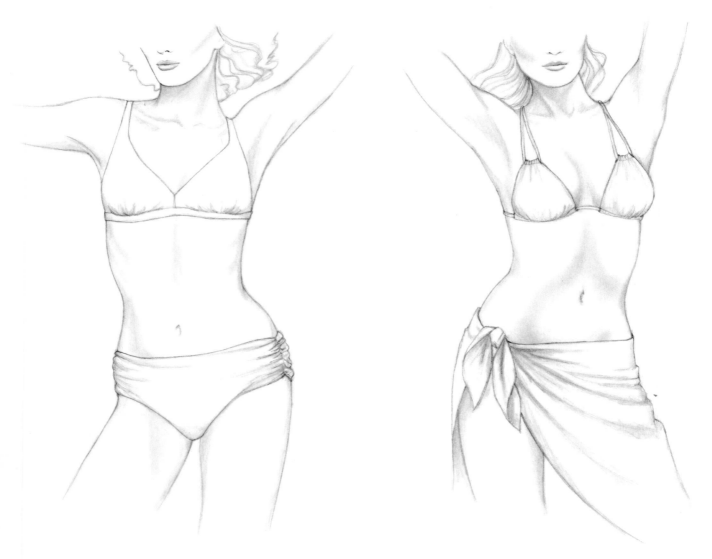

THE SEARCH FOR THE IDEAL BATHING SUIT

It's a rare woman who possesses a perfect figure. And it's an even rarer woman who thinks her figure is perfect. One of the sometimes disconcerting aspects of sunning is that sooner or later, one must reveal one's imperfections to the world.

The most practical way to deal with this is to select a flattering bathing suit. By flattering, we mean one that draws attention to your strong points while discreetly soft-pedaling your weak ones. Many suits do exactly this. Many other suits have an uncanny ability to make an actually quite nice figure look downright misshapen. The key to all this lies in understanding your own proportions. Herewith, some aspects to bear in mind.

Slim to the point of boniness. Soft materials—jersey, terrycloth, etc.—soften sharp edges. Horizontal stripes minimize the excessive narrowness of a very

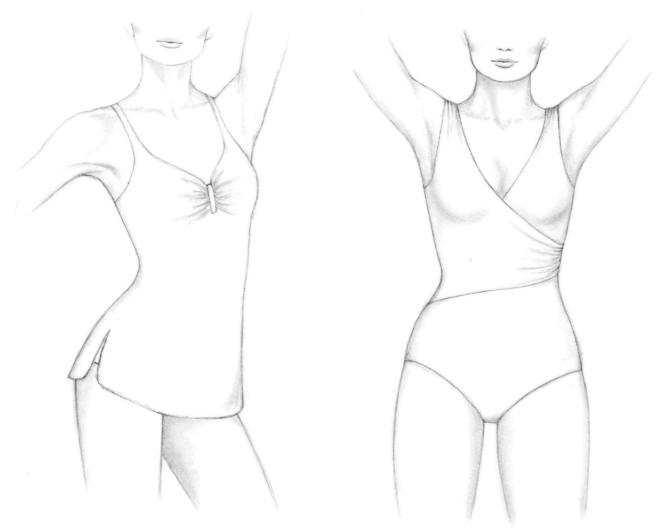

slender figure. If you like bikinis, try to get one with a bottom that rises at least high enough to cover the hipbone. If your bust is small, look for bikini tops with a little shirring at the center, or even an inner layer of fiberfill.

If you prefer a one-piece maillot, remember that a good deal of the effect depends on how the leg is cut. How high or how low can make all the difference in the world. Since it's impossible to generalize which height is for you, take our advice, and try on a variety of suits before deciding.

Bottom heavy. Bikinis do work on some bottom-heavy women, especially when they're adorned with a big, lightweight cotton scarf knotted around the waist. Called a *pareo*, this is a fashion popularized by resorts around the world.

Feel safer in a one-piece suit? Then try a leotard with enough gathering at the side to lead viewers' eyes away from problem thighs. Or a suit with a wraparound bodice for the same effect. Or a suit with a long torso and straight-hanging, open-sided skirt, which can be quite slenderizing. Whatever you do, don't put anything with a skirt onto your already wide hips.

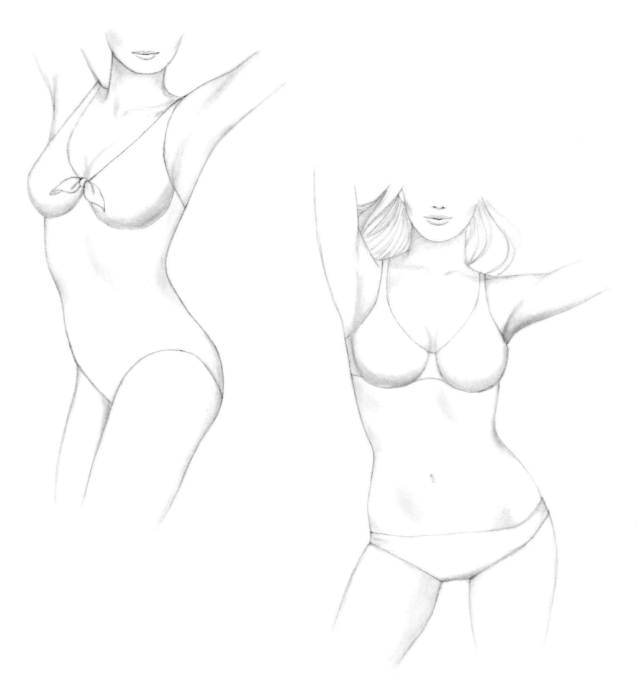

Top heavy. A heavy bust is usually more comfortable in a wired or shaped cup. Besides comfort, there's the minimizing effect to be considered, and the fact that the weight of an unsupported bosom can lead to unsightly strap marks on your shoulders.

You may very well be able to wear a bikini, but be sure to look for one not only with adequate bosom support, but also with a very low-waisted bottom. This low waist will give the figure a more balanced appearance.

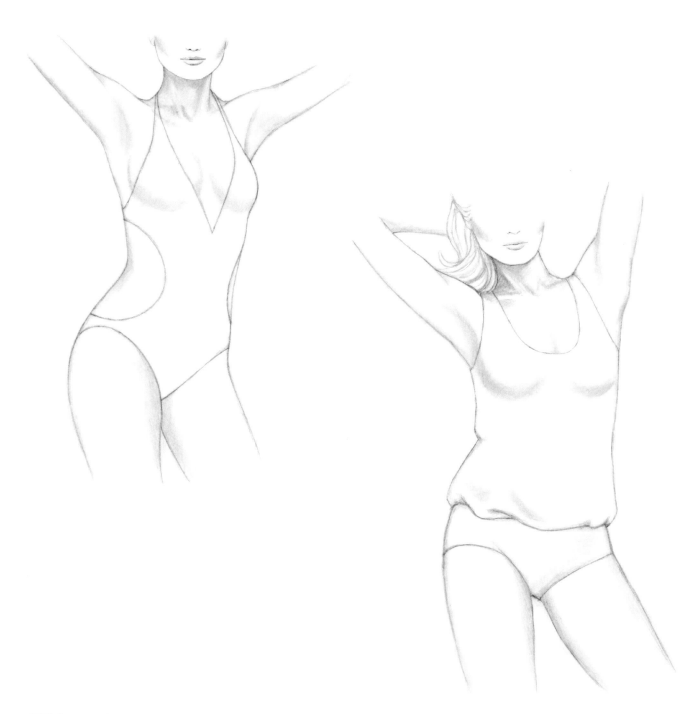

Thick waisted. You're best advised to stick with a one-piece suit, at least as far as promoting the illusion of a good figure. Such a suit, when cut away at the sides and/or plunged at the neckline, will further minimize your middle. And if your legs are good, a style that's cut high at the legline will also help. If you hate all of the above, there's always the blouson, which hides a wealth of imperfections.

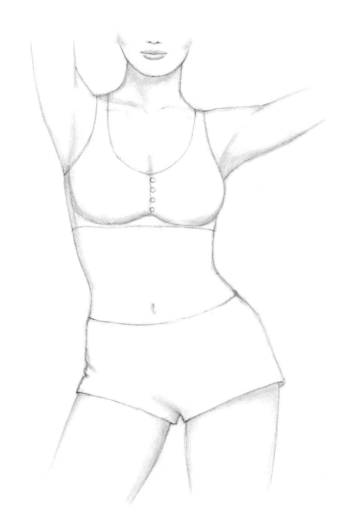

Well-proportioned, but heavy. A maillot or tank suit is always a good choice. If you have a nice flat tummy, you might also try a two-piece with either traditional bikini bottom or, if your upper leg is a little flabby, boy-leg styling.

6. Sunny Health: Exercise and Diet

The prospect of wearing a bathing suit brings the word "diet" immediately to mind. For many of us, that word conjures images of a sudden and radical departure from normal eating habits. Diets aren't perceived as much fun. And no small number of us crumble well before the diet has come anywhere close to achieving its stated goal, the elimination of unsightly excess poundage.

The problem with this view of things lies in the assumption that a sensible diet differs by definition from normal eating habits. The two *should* be the same. The best way to free yourself of unwanted weight, therefore, is not to gain it in the first place. The world teems with people who are naturally thin. They didn't get that way through endless starvation diets. Nor do they have weird glands or esoteric metabolisms. They simply don't overeat.

There's nothing mysterious about eating a properly balanced, naturally nourishing, and nonfattening diet, especially for those of us who live in the developed nations of the world. Although diet is the target of numerous fads and dubious assertions, balanced meals for most people require nothing more than eating reasonable daily amounts (measured in calories) of each of the major food groups. In other words, if you include protein, starch, greens, a bit of fat or oil, and water in every day's menu, you'll easily provide yourself with a balanced diet.

Every month of the year, magazines around the world publish strange non-nourishing diets whose collective purpose is abrupt weight loss. We don't believe in these diets. Furthermore, we refuse to jump on a bandwagon already crowded with apple diets and grapefruit diets and water diets and chocolate sundae diets and so on and so forth, *ad nauseam*. As far as we're concerned, these sorts of diets are part of the problem of overweight, not part of the cure.

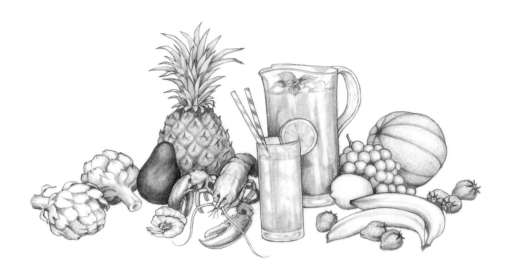

If you want a trim figure, you should start eating regular meals that aren't overly caloric. Results may come slowly, but they'll be long lasting. So instead of enduring constant inconveniences (as, for example, with diets that insist on a certain type of broiled fish that you know you'll never find in your neighborhood) or dubious nutrition (as with diets that totally exclude various food groups), our advice is to learn about calories.

CALORIE COUNTING: THE SAFE, SURE SYSTEM

All foods contain energy that can be measured in terms of the amount of heat produced when the food itself is burned. The unit measure of this heat is called a calorie, and it will accurately indicate exactly how much energy there is in every sort of food. Your body burns food in order to supply itself with energy. Calories not burned by the body are stored away as fat. It should therefore be fairly clear that the fatty tissue on any body simply represents the excess of calories consumed over those burned in the course of daily living.

Gaining control of your daily caloric intake first requires a knowledge of the caloric content of all the foods you eat. This task, simple as it is, often discourages people. But learning calories is far simpler than, say, learning a language. And besides, it's just one of those things that everybody should know. The best—really the only—way to learn is to get yourself a calorie book. Small abridged volumes are available in almost any good pharmacy. In addition, you should get a larger volume for more extensive reference and keep it in your kitchen. Carry your drugstore booklet with you at all times, and always remember to look up those items not included in the pocket guide in your bigger reference volume as soon as you get home. It won't take long to learn by heart the caloric content of nearly every food you eat. You'll also be able soon enough to estimate easily and accurately the caloric content of foods not contained in your books. It's merely a matter of patience.

To learn calories is useless, however, unless you know how to apply that knowledge. The trouble with most calorie diets is their attempt to be overly restrictive. 1000 calories per day, for instance, is ridiculously low. It's no wonder that people on such diets despair and go off them before they get results. Who can blame them? They're starving to death!

The key to weight loss—which we're going to call maintenance of desirable weight from now on—is knowing how to translate desirable weight into a specific number of daily calories necessary to maintain that weight. There is an old rule of thumb that works fairly well. Multiply your desirable weight by 15 and the result will be the number of daily calories necessary to maintain that weight.

Here now is a simple chart that contains desirable weight levels for women of varying heights. The lower weight in each case is for women with light frames; similarly, the upper weight is more appropriate for those with heavier frames.

Take this chart, locate your height, determine your approximate ideal weight, multiply that figure by 15, and the result will be the number of calories you will require each day in order to achieve that weight—and to stay there.

HEIGHT	DESIRABLE WEIGHT
5′ – 5′2″	95 – 110 lbs.
5′2″ – 5′4″	105 – 120 lbs.
5′4″ – 5′6″	110 – 130 lbs.
5′6″ – 5′8″	120 – 140 lbs.
5′8″ – 5′10″	125 – 145 lbs.
5′10″ – 6′	140 – 160 lbs.

You might find it both interesting and informative to multiply your current weight by 15 just to see how many calories you're consuming at present. The answer may surprise you. It doesn't take all that many extra calories to result in unattractive flab. And by the same token, to lose that extra flesh may not require as much self-denial as you think. Just limit yourself to the proper calorie intake level—and be patient.

If you're going to adopt this system, then do so with the intention of making it a lifetime commitment. Believe us, it's not hard to eat well and still not exceed your calorie limit. If you do exceed it, well then, cut back a little on the next day's calories. As long as your three-day average is in order, calorie limitation of this sort will insure maintenance of a desirable weight level.

Other helpful thoughts on weight maintenance:

1. Weigh yourself every day at the same time. There's no other way to accurately keep track.

2. Count (or estimate) the calories in every single thing that passes your lips. A few raisins here, a cookies there, a bite of somebody's burger, a glass of wine, they all add up (to about 230 calories just in these examples!).

3. Eat slowly.

4. Try to learn how to substitute low-cal foods for high-cal varieties. Diet soda or mineral water beats sugar-sweetened soft drinks by miles; fish or chicken contain far fewer calories than equivalent weights of red meat; white wine has only about two thirds the calories of red wine; certain donuts and crullers are much lighter than others, and often every bit as satisfying.

5. Forecast the day's meals *ahead of time.* Try to avoid—or at least be prepared for—situations of extreme temptation.

6. Limit the amount of food you keep around the house to just what you plan to prepare at mealtime.

EXERCISE AND THE BODY BEAUTIFUL

Calories are the key to maintenance of proper weight levels. Exercise is not. Exercise is great for toning muscles, increasing endurance, enhancing the grace of normal movement, flushing the complexion, improving balance, stimulating circulation, and contributing to an overall feeling of health and vitality. These are all excellent reasons to undertake a regular exercise program. But please, don't start exercising in order to lose weight.

It's not that exercise won't burn up calories. It will, and it will also burn them up faster than simply standing still. What's more, even strenuous exercise will not noticeably increase the appetite. But for all that, there just aren't enough calories burned even in the course of vigorous activities for the exercise itself to completely substitute for calorie control.

Having said that, we will again stress that exercise is a highly desirable thing. Making it a regular part of your life is much the same as adopting the caloric method of dietary control. It's not something to be alternately picked up and dropped as the mood strikes you. Exercise, unlike calories, can't be stored away. The benefits that accrue from regular jogging, tennis playing, or any other aerobic (meaning oxygenating) sport are temporary. Remain inactive for a week, even if you've been religiously working out for a month beforehand, and the toning and conditioning benefits you achieved will essentially vanish. So, if you determine to take up an exercise of some sort—be it running, tap dancing, tennis, squash, skiing, or whatever—you'll have to make it a part of every single week's activities. To be effective at all, there's no getting around it: Exercise must be done daily or every other day at least.

Different types of exercises have distinctly different purposes. Aerobic exercises, mentioned above, seek to elevate the rates of the respiratory and circulatory systems. Running is the prototypical aerobic exercise. It gets the blood pumping and fills the lungs with oxygen. Soon the whole body is filled with energizing oxygen. The muscular system is also toned, endurance is markedly improved, even mental breakthroughs are claimed to stem from well-oxygenated brains. Anything you do that gets you breathing hard and perspiring freely, and is sustained for at least twenty minutes will be aerobic. Runners' bodies also tend to develop a rather more pleasing conformation. They just look better put-together. But it's something that requires a real commitment and a minimum number of hours (approximately 4) per week.

Isometric exercises build muscles by pitting them against immovable objects. They do nothing to improve grace or suppleness, nor do they improve cardiovascular function. All they do is increase the size of your muscles. And as such, they're probably not what you're looking for.

Isotonic exercises, also known as gymnastics, develop strength and flexibility. Ballet and modern dance, yoga, and a myriad of specific muscle exercises (of the sort described below) fall into this category. These are just as valuable as aerobic exercises in promoting the grace and appearance of summer bodies.

Our advice would be to definitely adopt *some* kind of exercise program— and the sooner the better. Exercised bodies are naturally more attractive, if only because they move better. We're fans of aerobic exercises, but if running leaves you cold, we have ten recommended isotonic routines perfectly tailored for toning summer muscles. About half are designed to be done in a pool, the rest on dry land. To seriously embark on an isotonic routine of this sort means setting aside at least 15 to 20 minutes a day. Determine a sequence of exercises—any sequence will do—go through them all, then repeat the sequence until your 20 minutes is up.

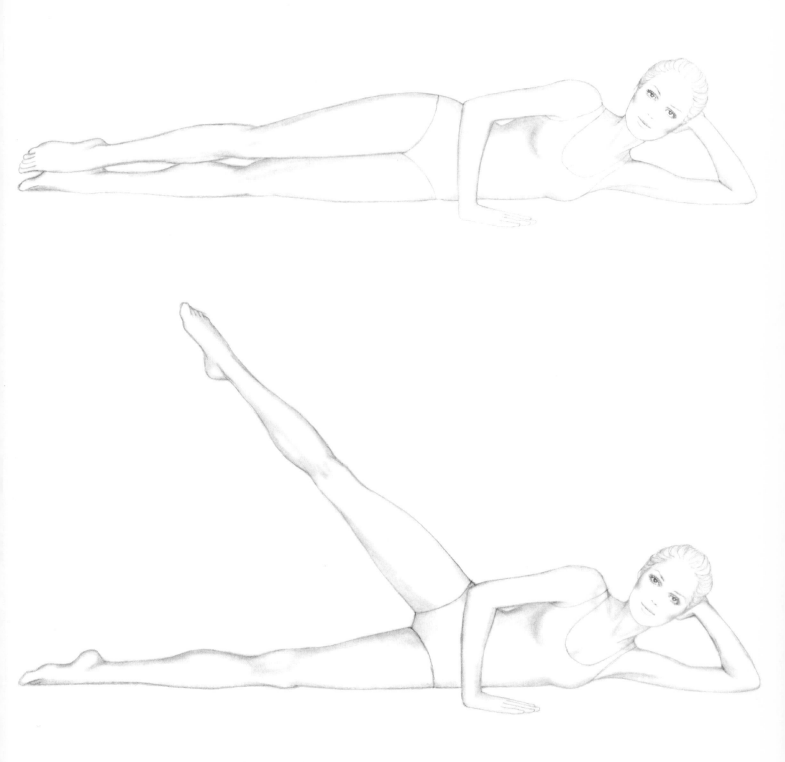

Leg raises. Lie on your side, head propped up on your arm. Use your free arm for balance. Point the toes down and slowly raise the upper leg as high as you can, then slowly let it down. Do this 10 times, then turn over and repeat with the other leg.

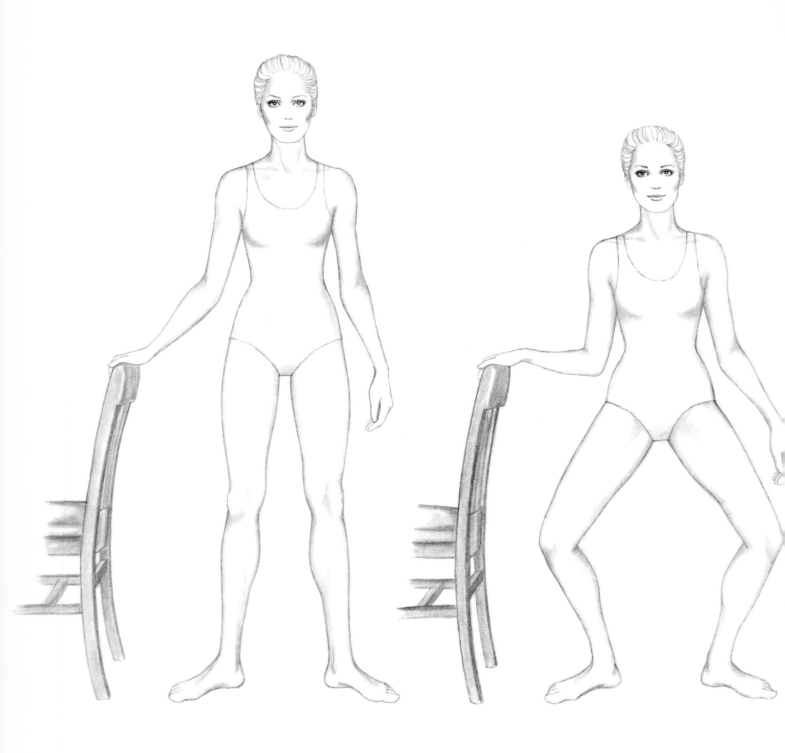

Knee bends. Stand with the feet slightly apart and facing out. Bend both knees, keeping the back straight, the head up, and the pelvis forward. Move slowly, so as to get maximum benefits in the thigh area. Start with 5 times and work up to 20.

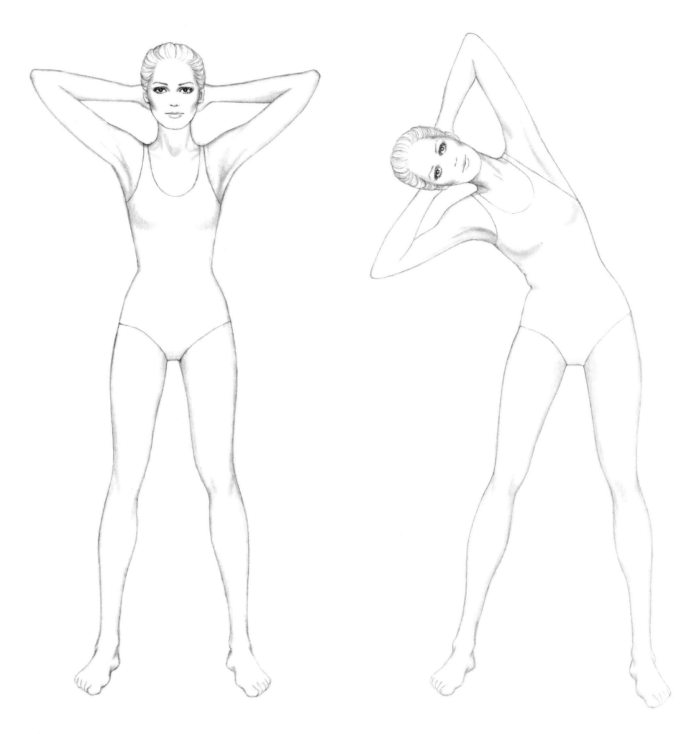

Waist arch. Hands behind the head, feet apart and firmly placed, knees unlocked, bend to the left and then to the right. Repeat this 20 times. For added suppleness, bend forward and swing the torso 360 degrees in one direction, then back around the other way, being sure to keep the feet in one position throughout. Repeat the torso swing 4 times.

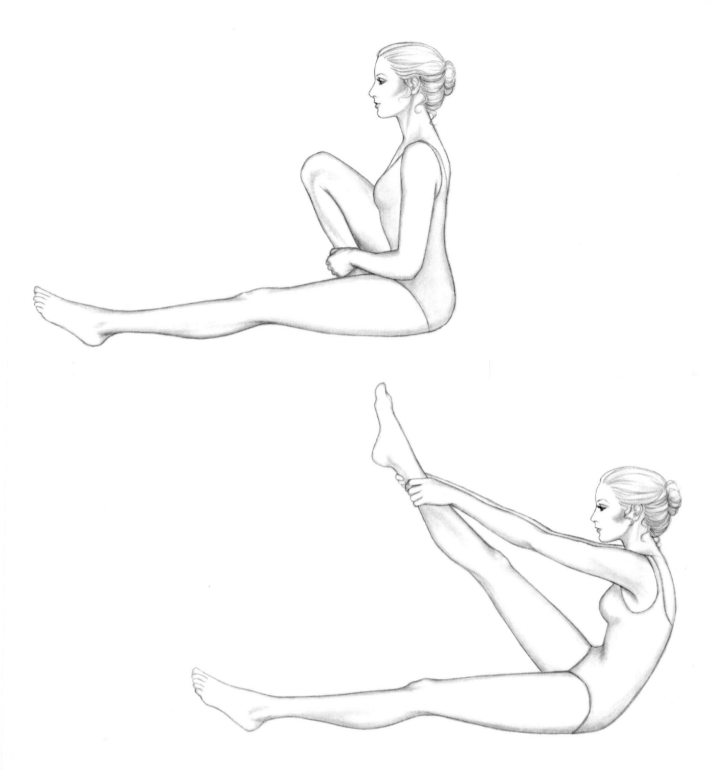

Leg stretch. Sit on the floor, left leg straight, right leg bent and held at the ankle. Then swing the right leg high—still holding the ankle—and keep it up there for a count of 3 before bringing it back to lowered position. Repeat 3 times, then switch legs.

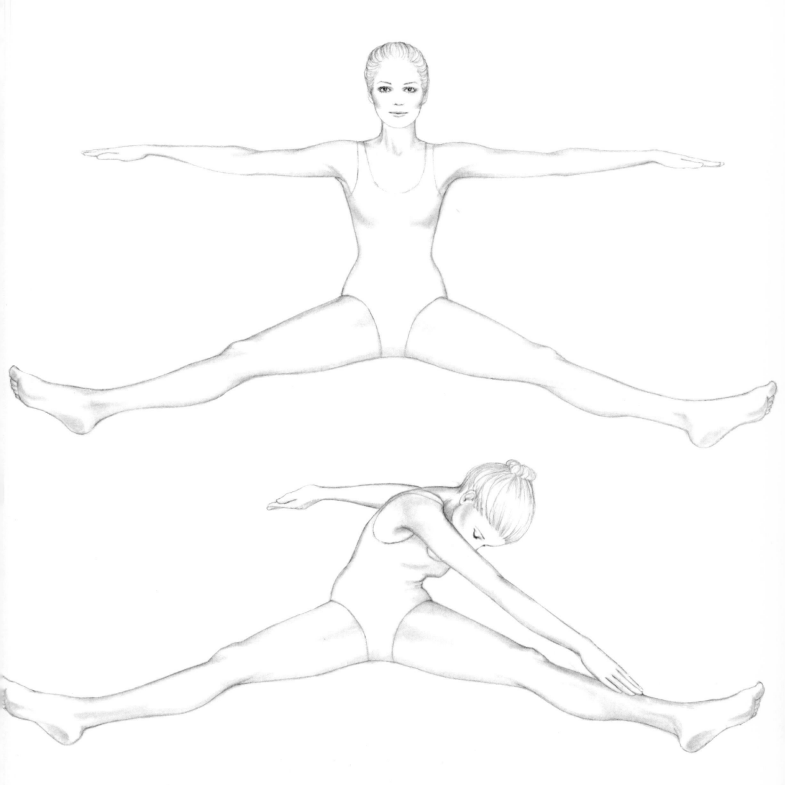

Toe touching. Sit upright on the floor, arms outstretched, legs apart. Swing rhythmically forward, and touch the right foot with the left hand. Sit back up, and then touch the left foot with the right hand. Repeat 20 times.

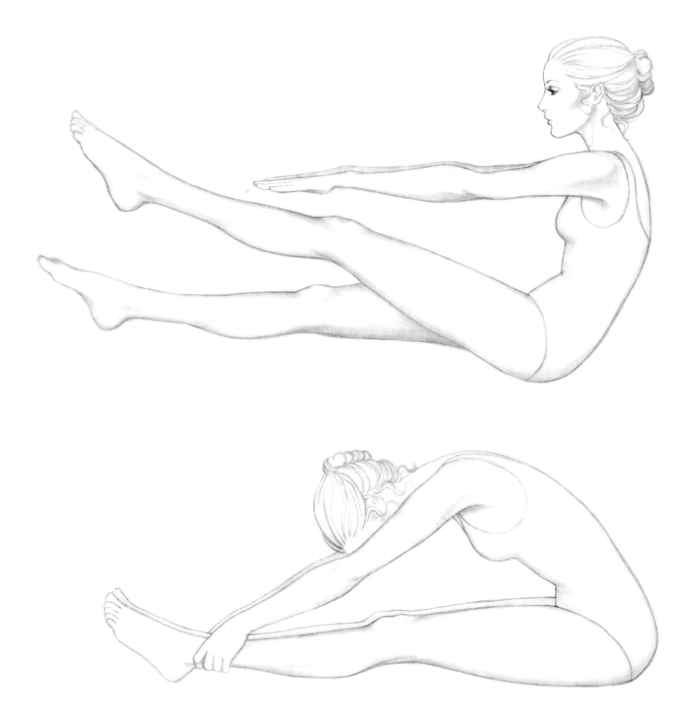

Abdomen toning. Sit upright with legs extended, and lean back, raising both legs off the floor. Lift your right leg higher than your left, then lower that leg and lift the left higher than the right, all the time keeping both legs elevated while you slowly kick them in the air. Do 6 kicks with each leg, then lower both to the floor, lean down, and, grasping the ankles, try to touch your head to your knees.

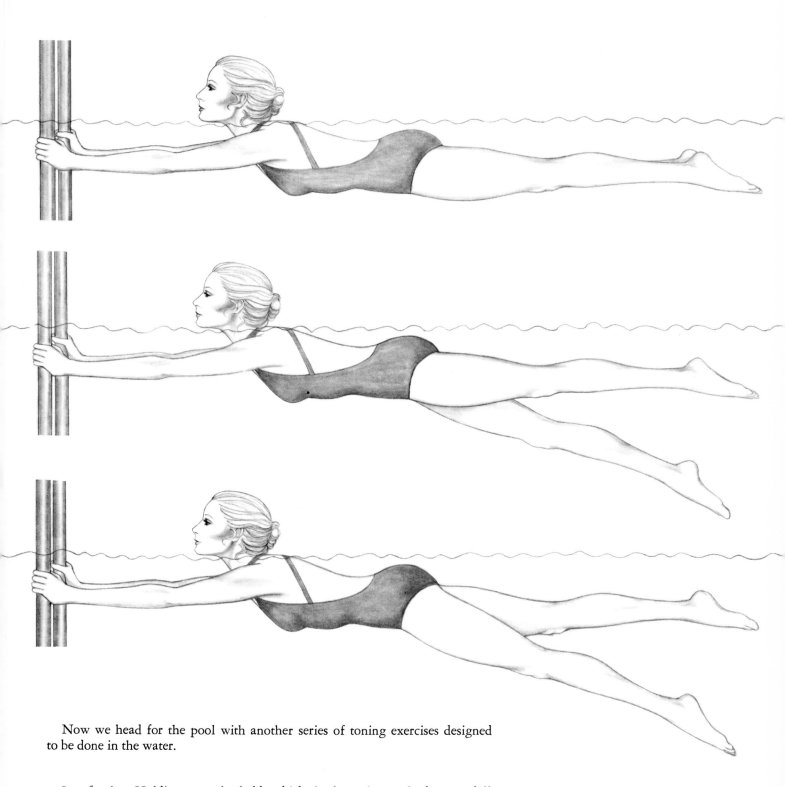

Now we head for the pool with another series of toning exercises designed to be done in the water.

Leg firming. Holding onto the ladder, kick the legs vigorously for two full minutes. Rest while you count to 20, and begin again. Repeat the cycle 3 times.

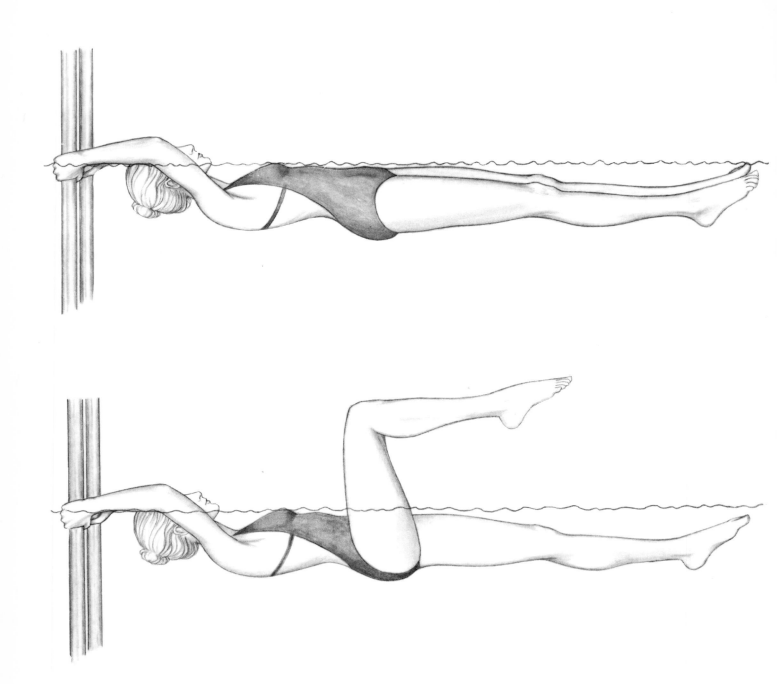

Abdomen and back. Float on your back, legs fully extended, arms outstretched over your head, grasping the ladder behind you. Keep your head back and your tummy tucked in—the secret of floating on top of the water, rather than fighting to stay parallel to the surface. Lift one leg, bending the knee at the same time until the thigh is at a right angle to your body, then return the leg to the outstretched position; repeat with the other leg. Repeat the cycle 10 times.

94

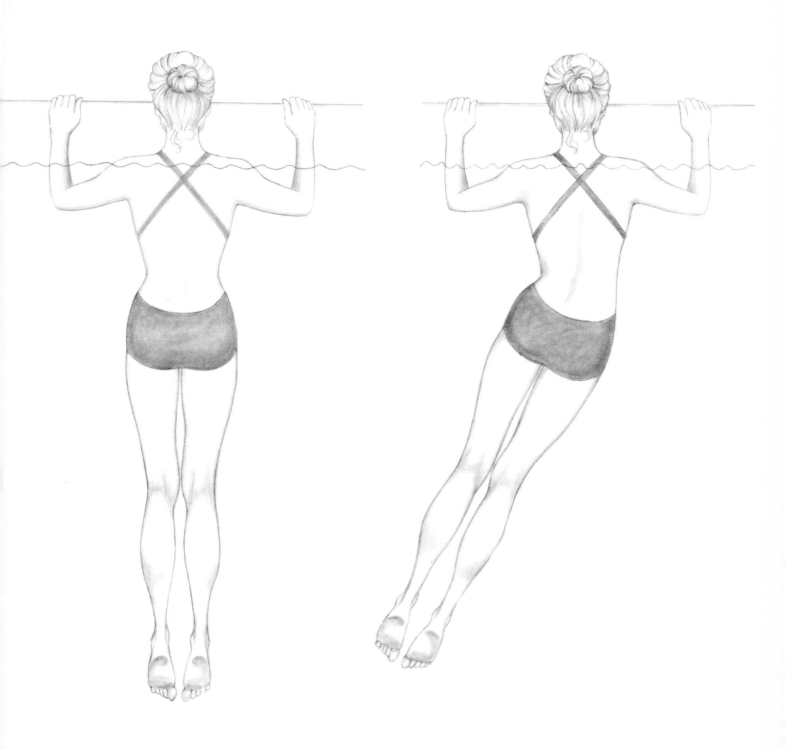

Waist and torso toning. Head for the deep water, face the side of the pool, and hold onto the edge. Point both feet straight down, then, bending at the waist, swing first to one side then to the other in a continuous motion. Keep it up for two minutes.

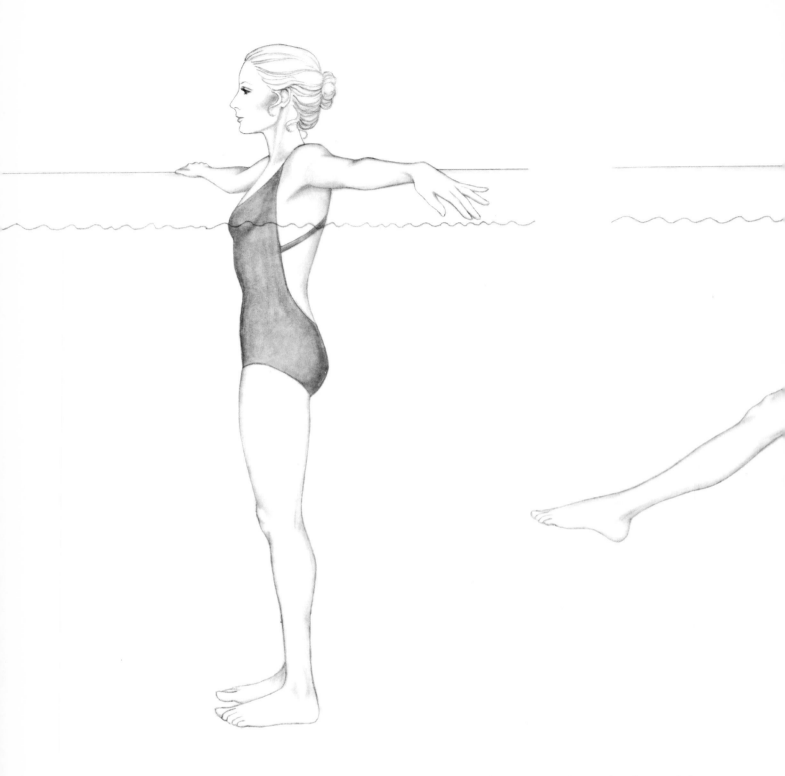

Waist slenderizing. Stand shoulder height in the pool and extend the arms. First swing the right leg forward as far as possible, then backward as far as possible. Repeat with the left leg, do each leg 12 times.

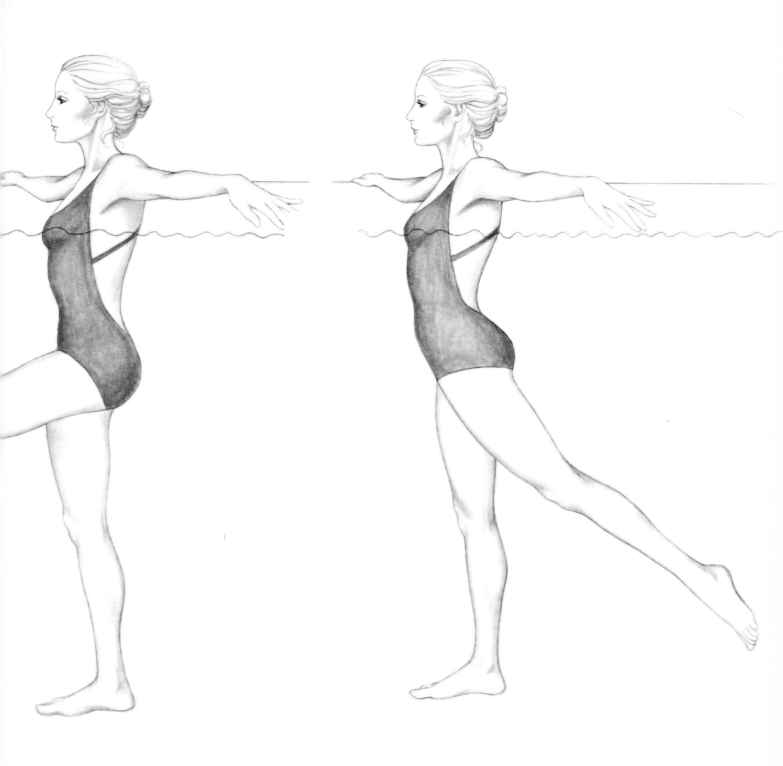

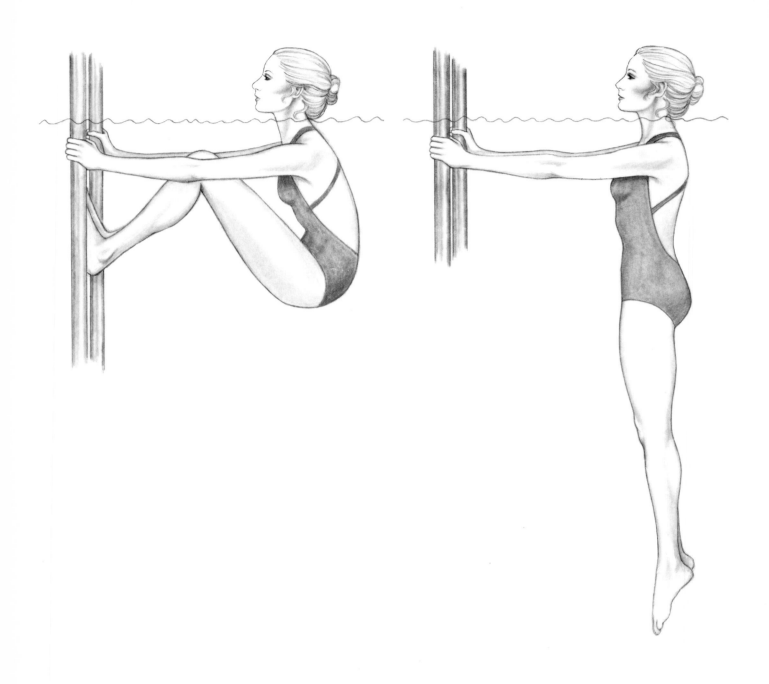

Abdomen and leg toning. Face the ladder, holding on with both hands, and draw the feet up as illustrated. Slowly lower the feet, first to a straight-down position, then to a prone position with the stomach facing the bottom of the pool. Make the motion as smooth as possible, then return to the original position. Work up to 25 times.

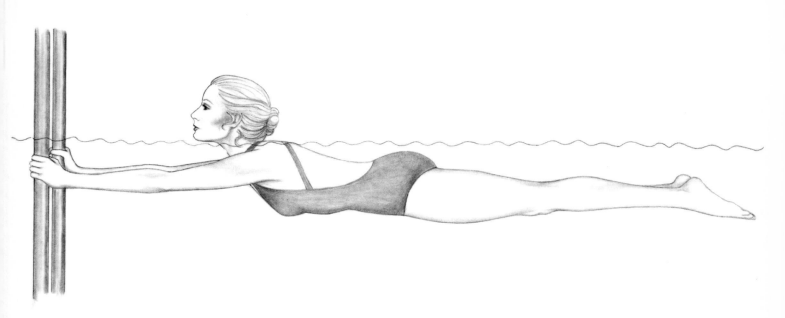

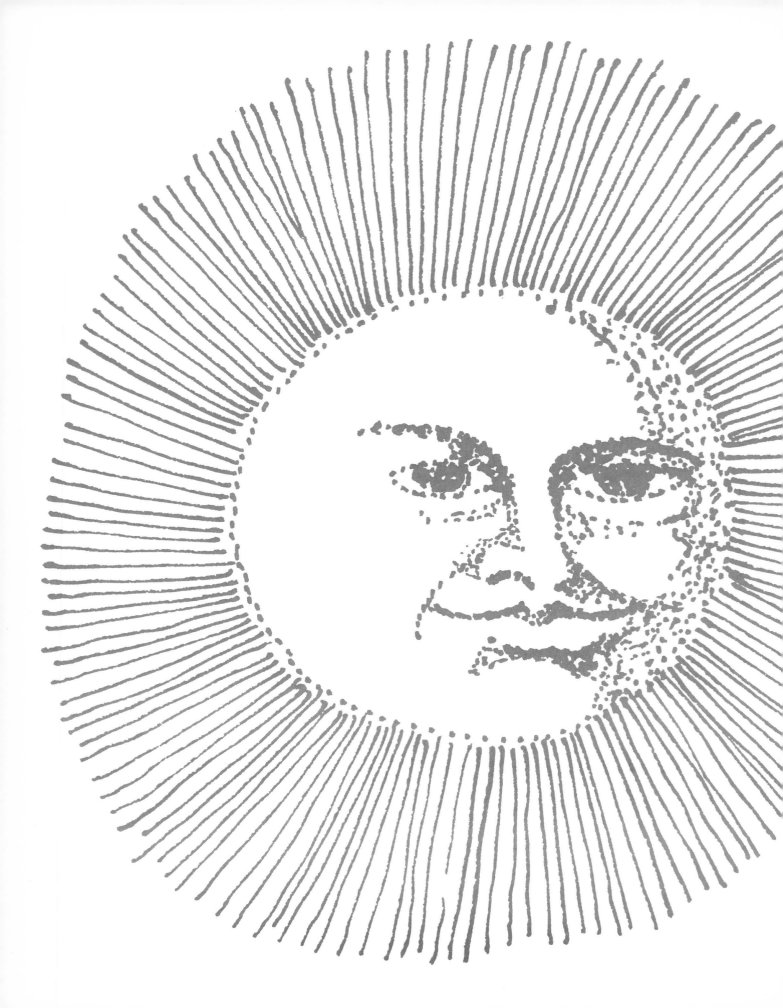

PART II
FACTS AND FUN
RE: THE SUN

One Norse tale tells of Frigga's struggle to protect her son Balder and ensure him of eternal life. In the end she fails, and the saga of Balder recounts his death at the hands of his blind brother, Hoder, god of night, who is tricked into slaying Balder with a spear of mistletoe, the one substance in the Norse universe over which light cannot prevail.

SYMBOLS AND CEREMONIES

Fueled by such natural and terrorizing phenomena as eclipses, dust storms, and clouds of volcanic smoke—not to mention long stretches of sunless weather —the fear and awe of the sun inspired such sophisticated structures as Stonehenge, now generally recognized to have been a vast solar calendar that predicted the life of the sun for an apprehensive Druid civilization. Similar concerns inspired the Sumerians to develop astronomy, albeit a system befuddled by astrology. And it inspired the Chinese to such accurate observations of the skies that they were able to record sun spots. The plains Indians of North America danced their obeisance to the sun, and among some groups, tribal leaders prostrated themselves in noontime ceremonies, slashing themselves with knives, praying to take on all the sins of the people so the sun would not halt its daily journey. Complex mystical ceremonies proliferated throughout the primitive and ancient worlds—a great number of them organized around the triangle and the swastika, virtually universal symbols for the sun and its earthly secondary power, fire. Egyptians used the triangle as model for the pyramids, but tombs and monuments in pyramidal form appeared as far away as China, Java, and Central America.

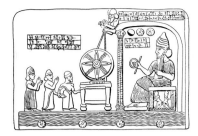

Shamash, the Sumerian sun god, had to overcome cosmic obstacles to assure the continuance of light from year to year.

The eerie grandeur of the Stonehenge Monoliths is a testimony to the enormous energy and ingenuity that human beings have devoted to worshiping and harnessing the sun's power. The careful arrangement of these stones seems to suggest that the Druids used Stonehenge as an elaborate solar calendar.

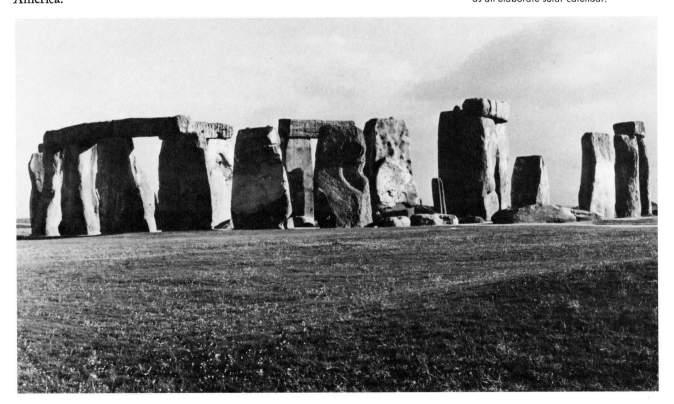

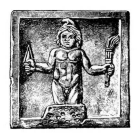

Mithra, a Persian sun god, seen here with a torch in one hand and a sword in the other, was believed to have been born from solid rock. The rock, representing darkness, was cast off by the power of the lighted torch (the sun).

THE SUN IN JUDEO–CHRISTIAN TRADITION

Fear and awe of the sun persisted, not only from culture to culture, but from century to century. Gods of the sun were among those Moses railed against when he discovered the children of Israel praying to graven images and clinging to the old polytheistic myths of ancient Egyptian and Mesopotamian cultures. The tale of Samson may derive from one such solar myth. His famous locks of hair, scholars point out, possibly comparable to the rays of the sun, are shorn by Delilah, whose name may derive from *lilah*, the Hebrew word for night. Thus Samson loses his strength in her arms, recovering it for one more feat when his hair grows again, just as the sun rises for one more round.

Centuries later, around 400 A.D., the Christians had to contend with the suddenly popular Mithra, a latter-day sun god of the Persians. Roman soldiers had embraced the cult, celebrating the birth of the sun god, as they had the Saturnalia, at the winter solstice—complete with feasting and gift-giving. The Christian victory came when they too incorporated the gifting and feasting into their annual festival and moved Christmas to that time of year when the sun stops its annual descent and begins its rise in the heavens once again. We ourselves approach the twenty-first century, and the Christian world still lights up each year with a festival that once celebrated, not the birth of the Son of God, but the birth of Mithra, god of the sun.

We still worship the sun, of course. Today, he's God of the Tan, and the contemporary monuments we construct for him are likely to be solar energy collectors. Although many of the fears of those primitive watchers of the sky have been dispelled by modern astronomy, science has confirmed their most terrifying surmise—the belief that one day, indeed, the sun will die.

8. Facts Re:The Sun

Most astronomers agree that the universe itself was born about 15–20 billion years ago, emerging mysteriously from the shattering explosion known as the Big Bang. No one knows what caused the Bang—it's the true miracle of creation. And the evidence suggests that we will never know. It's become generally accepted, though, that the universe had such a beginning and will have an end, in some impossibly distant future difficult to contemplate. As we'll see, the universe that gave birth to our sun will, someday, quietly note its passing.

ONE AMONG BILLIONS

The apparently remarkable star we call our sun is some 93 million miles away. If you booked passage on a rocket that zipped along at 25,000 mph, it would take you over five months to get there. A journey to the next nearest star, however, would take 300,000 times as long. You can begin to appreciate the sizes and distances involved if you think of the sun as a light bulb shining on top of the Eiffel Tower. The Earth is then a mosquito just across the street, and the next star is another light bulb, beaming atop a building somewhere near Stockholm. But, regardless of how the sun actually stacks up as a star by universal standards, it's the only one we've got.

What we've got is, to state it baldly, pretty ordinary—a middle-aged, average size star, with a rather typical glow. The sun that dazzles us with its apparently fierce radiance is what astronomers call a yellow dwarf, or fifth-magnitude star. The blue super-giant, Rigel, in the constellation Orion, shines 40,000 times more brightly. And while some stars are 10 times smaller, others are 1000 times as large. The red giant, Betelgeuse, for example, is only 350 times the size of

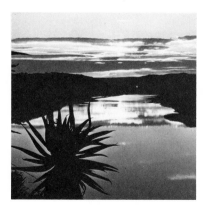

At sunset, a huge Aloe is reflected in the still waters of the Transkei, South Africa.

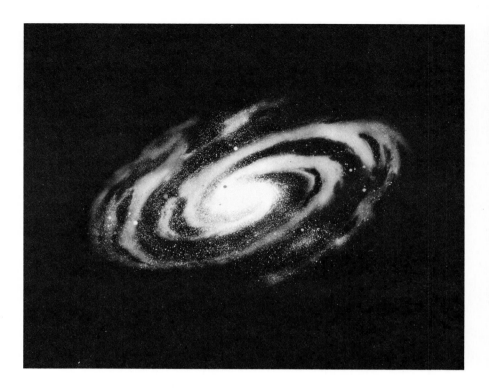

our sun. But if it were to take the sun's place in our solar system, Betelgeuse would engulf Mercury, Venus, the Earth, and Mars.

Even by galactic standards, our sun isn't very important. Our solar system of nine planets and assorted moons belongs to the galaxy known as the Milky Way. A galaxy is a localized cluster of stars, with dust and gas floating in between. Galaxies take different shapes. Ours is one of those that astronomers call spiral galaxies—shaped something like an oval cookie with curved arms projecting from several points along its edge. Our sun is but one of over 200 billion stars in the Milky Way alone. What's more, the universe is filled with groups of galaxies, each group containing from a few to a few hundred. In all, there are billions of galaxies, of which the Milky Way is not a very impressive specimen. But it, too, is the only one within reach. The light from Andromeda, our nearest galactic neighbor, takes two million years to reach us.

From the cosmic perspective, our sun, sitting in one of the Milky Way's spiral arms, about three-quarters of the way out from the galaxy's center, becomes in the words of one uncharitable observer, "an inconsequential light-speck lost on the outskirts of a minor galaxy."

SOME VITAL STATISTICS

If the sun is only average from the universal perspective, the view from Earth is awesome. So vast is the cosmos that astronomers deal as a matter of course with numbers so large as to slip beyond our ability to really grasp them. But the accumulated weight of the frequent billions, trillions, even octillions needed to describe solar phenomena can't fail to stagger Earth-bound imaginations.

A celestial globe, 5 feet in diameter, illustrated a treatise by Tycho Brane. Great progress in astronomy during the sixteenth century benefited navigation in the years of discovery.

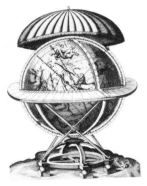

The sun's diameter is about 865,000 miles—109 times bigger than Earth's, 400 times bigger than the moon's. Its volume, roughly 335 quadrillion cubic miles, is 1,300,000 times that of Earth.

The sun is a mass of 2 billion, billion, billion tons of gases. That accounts for 99.8 percent of the mass of the entire solar system—333,000 times the Earth's mere 6.6 sextillion tons, 1047 times the mass of Jupiter, the largest planet. By this standard, the planets and their various moons are little more than a rather fine space debris—dust flicked off the shoulder of the sun.

This solar mass creates a gravitational pull 28 times that on Earth. If you're a trim 120 pounds down here, you'd tip the scales at a rather sluggish 3368 in a solar weigh-in. The enormous gravity is, however, what keeps the sun in shape. It pulls inward with a force that precisely counterbalances the outward push of the expanding gases, so it keeps the sun from simply flying apart.

A few hundred years ago, we learned, much to our chagrin, that the Earth is not the fixed point and center of the universe. Neither is the sun, of course. For while we and the rest of the solar system do revolve around the sun, the sun is far from motionless. Like the Earth, it revolves on an axis, roughly once a month. But because it's gaseous rather than solid, with considerable wavelike turbulence on the surface, the sun's rotation is uneven. Layers of gas near the solar equator complete one full rotation every 27 days. Near the poles, they take 31 days or more. We've also learned, much more recently, that our entire galaxy rotates around its center. The arm of the Milky Way that contains our sun and solar system completes one majestic celestial revolution every 250 million years.

THE SOURCE: HEAT AND LIGHT FROM THE SUN

Because the Earth's orbit around the sun is elliptical, or oval-shaped, our distance from the sun varies from about 91.4 to 94.5 million miles. At the average distance of 93 million miles, the light and heat energy reaching Earth take 8 minutes and 20 seconds to get here, traveling at the speed of light—186,282 miles per second. While changes in weather and other conditions in the Earth's atmosphere make the apparent heat and brightness of the sun vary, it is actually emitting a thoroughly constant glow equal to 2.5 billion, billion, billion candles—millions of billions of billions of watts.

Temperatures at the sun's core reach 27 million degrees Fahrenheit, drop to as low as 7700 degrees in the sun's inner atmosphere, then rise again to nearly 5.5 million degrees in the outer atmosphere. But the solar radiation that arrives on Earth has an energy equivalent to 126 watts per square foot, and produces temperature changes in a range only slightly greater than 100 degrees. Although this solar energy has, of course, been sufficient to sustain life on our planet, it represents a mere one two-billionth of the total energy radiating from the sun. All the rest is lost in space.

THE THERMONUCLEAR FURNACE

Solar radiations are the end-products of thermonuclear reactions at the sun's core. Like the rest of the universe, our sun is composed of 74 percent hydrogen, and almost 25 percent helium. Of the other 90 natural elements, scientists have detected traces of 68 in the remaining 1–2 percent of the sun's matter.

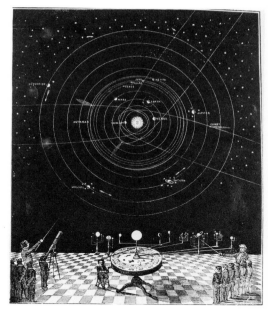

By the nineteenth century, our knowledge of the solar system, while growing, was still clearly imperfect. The asteroids that orbit the sun between Mars and Jupiter had been identified, but the relative distances of the planets, particularly Saturn, Uranus (Herschel), and Neptune (Leverrier) had been badly underestimated, and Pluto had not yet been discovered.

Inside the flaming sun, layers of molten rocks, gases, and volatile sub-atomic particles provide fuel for our solar system's most efficient furnace. The chromosphere (A) filters out some of the harshest radiation that is created when material from the core (E) and the radiative zone (D) undergoes fusion and is thrown out through the convective zone (C) and transitional region, into the darkness of space.

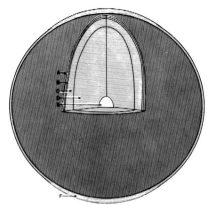

The solar halo, caused by flares leaping many thousands of miles out from the sun's surface, is seen here from an altitude of about 6,000 feet, filtered through a layer of cirro-stratus clouds.

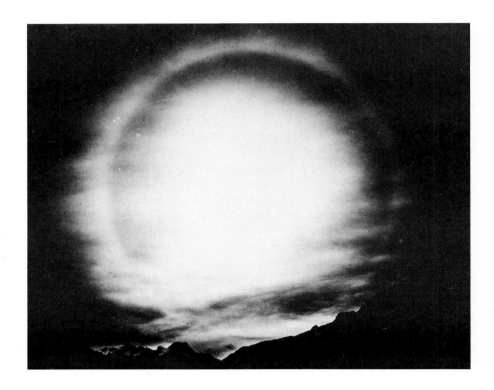

The shadow created by the central rod, or "gnomon" of this sundial, shows that it is almost high noon. For the reading to be accurate, the "gnomon" must point due north and angle between gnomon and the face must be equal in degrees to the degrees of latitude at the sundial's location.

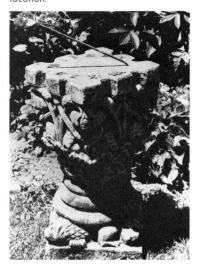

In the furnace of the sun's core, under pressures equal to a billion Earth atmospheres, protons of hydrogen atoms fuse together in a multistep process that creates helium atoms plus energy. *Every second*, this nuclear fusion burns up *4 million tons* of hydrogen, releasing energy equivalent to a trillion hydrogen bombs, in 100 trillion, trillion, trillion individual fusion reactions.

The sun's nuclear energy is carried in little packets called photons, which form waves that begin moving away from the core out toward the sun's surface. Most of this primary radiation quickly takes the form of gamma rays, which, if released raw at the sun's surface, would destroy everything in their path. Fortunately, the photons in the gamma rays must fight their way through almost 400,000 miles of churning solar gases. During this journey, they are constantly colliding with the protons, electrons, and other particles that comprise the atoms of solar gases—a process that defuses the enormous destructive energy of gamma rays, converting it into waves of the various other types of radiation that comprise what is called the electromagnetic spectrum. These waves include X rays, ultraviolet rays, visible light, infrared rays, microwaves, radio waves, and electric current.

The nature and characteristics of each type of radiation are determined by the amount of energy in its photons. The countless billions of collisions of gamma photons, in which their energy is continually absorbed and reradiated in different forms, is the reason why most of what eventually reaches the sun's surface, or photosphere, has the photon energy characteristics of visible light. The remaining surface radiation, some of which could be extremely damaging to life on Earth, is further screened by the chromosphere and corona—the primary regions of the sun's atmosphere—and then again by various layers and radiation belts in the Earth's atmosphere.

The visible light that will creep over the horizon at sunrise tomorrow morning will take only eight and one-third minutes to get here from the sun's surface. But the light was created before the dawn of civilization and has taken nearly a million years to fight its way up from core to solar surface.

SOLAR EVENTS

The solar surface, as most of us know, becomes covered periodically with dark areas called sunspots—often up to hundred at a time—many of which are larger than the Earth itself. Sunspots tend to appear in groups. The number of groups usually peaks quickly, then fades slowly during sunspot cycles whose average length is eleven years, though some cycles have run as few as seven and as many as seventeen years. There have been some long periods of history with almost no sunspot activity at all, but the spots have been observed since the time of Galileo. When he and other seventeenth-century astronomers reported their telescopic observations of spots on the solar surface, the Church was extremely uneasy about the suggestion that the sun—the "perfect fire" made by the Creator—was blemished. Today we know that the blemishes are caused by enormous concentrations of magnetic force, which cool the solar surface and result in the darkening perceived as spots.

Sunspots themselves don't appear to have any particular effect on Earth. Most astronomers now refer to solar activity cycles, since sunspots are simply the most visible sign of a variety of related occurrences, all of which seem to stem from constant, extraordinary shifts in the sun's magnetic fields. These solar events include the hotspots known as faculae and plages; immense prominences of hot gas that can shoot hundreds of thousands of miles up into the sun's corona, or outer atmosphere; and solar flares—sudden cataclysms occurring in the vicinity of sunspots—that can explode with the force of a million atomic bombs, providing enough energy to satisfy the entire demand on Earth for 100,000 years.

Solar flares are believed to bear most of the responsibility for severe but brief radar and shortwave radio interference, certain electric power disruptions, breakdowns in wire communication networks, and the appearance of the aurora borealis, or northern lights. While there is some evidence to suggest that the eleven-year solar activity cycles have certain effects on human body chemistry, there are even stronger indications that the cycles affect such matters as the depth of the Earth's large lakes, the size of growth rings on trees, and the formation of cyclones and other weather abnormalities. It's even been suggested that the eleven-year cycle of great Burgundy vintages is no mere coincidence.

THE SUN AND WEATHER

The sun may give us tomorrow's power, but it gives us our weather today. The sun evaporates water in oceans, lakes, and rivers, which eventually falls back to earth as rain and snow. While this water is suspended in our atmosphere, it forms clouds, which reflect some sunlight back into space. This partial reflection, and the fact that the sun's rays strike the earth at varying angles during different seasons, combine to produce an uneven heating of the atmosphere. Differences in air pressure result, and as air masses move from high to low pressure areas, they create winds and bring weather changes.

The angle at which sunlight strikes—and not our distance from the sun—is also the main factor controlling temperature on Earth. In fact, when it's summer in the northern hemisphere, we're actually farther from the sun than we are in winter. But the tilt of the Earth's axis places us more directly beneath the sun's rays, which have less atmosphere to penetrate and thus create more heat. Think of a flashlight shining on a wall. The light is brighter at the center than at the edges, where the light rays have traveled further from the flashlight and strike the wall more obliquely. These same principles explain the relatively stable climates and steady temperatures found near the equator, where the tilt of the axis produces little change on the angles at which sunlight strikes.

THE DEATH OF THE SUN

If the sun stopped producing new energy tomorrow, we could live on in sublime ignorance for a million years. But it's not likely to do so. Most current estimates give the sun an additional lease on life of some 5 billion years. But it *will* die.

In a few billion years, the hydrogen supply at the core, which is being converted to energy at the phenomenal rate of 4 million tons a second, will run down sufficiently for the core to begin to contract. The contraction will drive temperatures up, increase the rate of fusion, and create outward pressures that will overcome the force of the sun's gravity. The sun will start to expand—its diameter increasing by millions of miles. It will expand until metals melt on Earth, and the oceans boil. It will expand until it swallows the Earth, Mars, and beyond. The sun will become a red giant.

After a few hundred million years in this stage of its life cycle, the solar gravity of this enormous sun will once more overcome the outward pressure of the turbulent gases, and contraction will set in once again. But without sufficient hydrogen to burn, this time the contraction won't be reversed. The red giant will continue to shrink, into a white dwarf—perhaps the size of its former planet, Earth. The dwarf will glow, increasingly feebly, for perhaps a billion years. Ultimately, the remaining heat and energy will be thoroughly exhausted, reducing the source, our splendid sun, to a blackened cinder. For all its fiery splendor, when the sun finally fades it will abdicate its kingly position in our universe, "not with a bang but a whimper."

9. Sun Signs

No book about the sun would be complete without a discussion of astrology, the ancient system of thought that assumes that celestial bodies influence human behavior, and which attempts to interpret that influence. As the sun is central to our lives—illuminating our days, warming us, nourishing our crops—so is it also the focus of astrological thinking, the blazing star around which the planets of our solar system revolve.

Just as the sun is the center of our solar system, these days it seems that astrology is the center of our social system. At social gatherings a remark like, "You must be a Capricorn," has, as ice-breaking conversation, become as commonplace as, "What do you do for a living?" Tabloid headlines scream: "Astrologer Predicts Starlet Will Marry." Nearly every newspaper and popular magazine offers a column with brief predictions for each of the twelve signs of the zodiac.

Whatever your attitude toward astrology—whether you won't make a move without consulting your horoscope, or whether you classify it in the realm of the ridiculous along with Ouija boards and patent medicines—you probably know your sun sign and read an occasional horoscope in the pages of your monthly fashion magazine. Astrology is an interesting and complex subject for study, with a long history and tradition. Our aim in this chapter is to clarify the basics of astrology for the casual horoscope reader, to help you understand what's behind these seemingly casual predictions, and perhaps add a new dimension to your cocktail party conversation and tabloid-reading!

A Celtiberian coin.

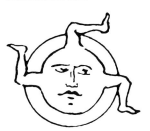

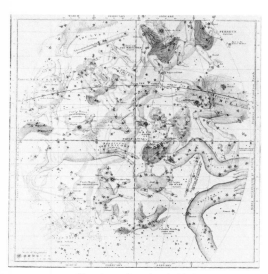

The winter sky, identifiable because of the presence of Orion, is shown with Gemini, Taurus, and Cancer, in this 1835 *Chart of the Heavens.*

A BRIEF HISTORY OF ASTROLOGY

We have always been stargazers. The vastness and the beauty of the stars and the constant brilliance of the sun have comforted, bewildered, and confused us. Astrology, in its basic form, evolved as our first attempt to explain what was going on in the universe. We noted that Orion (or the group of stars that came to be called Orion) appeared only in the winter; we saw that the sun seemed to go around the earth once a day; we made observations of the heavens—some correct, some way off the mark—and from such observations we tried to forge an explanation of our physical environment.

As time passed, man's observations and interpretations became more and more complicated. Information about the movement of the planets and changes in visible constellations and the weather—and how they all seemed to affect people's actions and personalities—became part of a body of knowledge that was passed from one generation to the next.

Western astrologers believe that their science existed in this rudimentary state before the dawn of civilization.* Astrological records were first kept, however, by the Chaldeans. This ancient people lived approximately 2500 years ago in the Tigris-Euphrates valley, where the dry, cloudless climate was ideal for observing and identifying many of the constellations and fixed stars.

Numerous references are made to astrology in the Old Testament, where astrologers are referred to as "Chaldeans"—a term later adopted by the Greeks and Romans—and the twelve tribes of Israel are each associated with a sign of the zodiac.

When Assyria conquered the Babylonian empire, of which the Chaldeans' land was a part, Babylonian lore was absorbed into Assyrian culture. Astrology had spread to Egypt by the sixth century B.C., and a few hundred years later, to Greece. In the second century B.C., practicing astrologers appeared as far away as Rome. By the second century A.D., astrology had evolved to the point where it was similar to the form in which we know it today.

The advent of Christianity focused much attention, both favorable and critical, on astrology. Some early Christians accepted astrology, citing the Star of the Nativity as an astrological sign; in some early Christian art Christ is portrayed as a sun god. But most Christians rejected astrology as immoral. In 323 A.D., when Constantine became emperor of Rome and legalized Christianity, astrology fell into disfavor. It did not die out, however, but merely went underground.

From the sixth to the ninth centuries, records of astrological studies in Western Europe are rare. Around 1000 A.D., there was a limited revival in Baghdad, now the capital of Iraq. Because of this renaissance and the general spread of Islamic culture, astrology reached Spain. But it wasn't until 1200 that astrology was again widely studied. Records of this time indicate that the first chancellor of Oxford University regarded astrology, or astronomy (the two were then the same), as the "supreme science." During the Middle

---

* Astrology has flourished both in Eastern and Western cultures, although in different forms. The old civilizations of South America and Mexico had astrological systems, as did China and India. It is in India, in fact, where astrology, which incorporates the concept of reincarnation, currently has its greatest popularity. But the astrological system that prevails in the Western world had its roots in the Middle East.

114

Ages, Italy was fertile ground for astrological study, which was accepted in some form by the Catholic Church.

Since the Middle Ages, astrology has gone in and out of vogue. But its study, commentaries on it, and references to it in literature have grown with every generation.

HOW THE SYSTEM OF ASTROLOGY WORKS

Astrological interpretations are made by noting the positions of the sun, moon, planets, stars, and asteroids and determining their relationship to the Earth and each other at specific times and in specific locations during our lives.

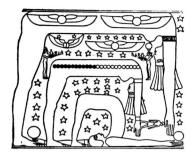

The Egyptians imagined that the Cosmos was defined by the Sun Goddess who oversaw the rising and setting sun, the stars, and the earth.

The position of these heavenly bodies is believed to exert a strong effect on each individual on Earth. The exact nature of that effect is determined by the unique arrangement of the cosmos at the moment of birth. As you will see, everyone responds differently to the same daily cosmic arrangements because the daily order is felt in relationship to one's unique birth order.

Astrologers assert that their function is to offer us insight into our basic temperament, personality traits, weaknesses, strengths, and the course of our past, present, and future life. But how can a stargazer translate her observations of the cosmos into astrological calculations and interpretations? Let's look at the process of "reading the heavens."

HOW DO WE DETERMINE THE POSITION OF THE STARS?

In order to find out how we have been affected by the cosmos, we need to analyze the position of the heavenly bodies at our time of birth or during a specific incident in our lives. For example, let's say you had a bad day last week (forgot your keys, fought with your friends, got a traffic ticket). You can find out what part the cosmos played in your fortunes. First, pinpoint the specific day and hour when your bad luck began. Second, pinpoint the location. Third, consult an ephemeris. An ephemeris is a book of charts that gives the location of all the important heavenly bodies, in many locations, at all times, far into the past and future. Those localities that are not specifically mentioned can be easily determined by figuring out the difference in latitude between the nearest locale mentioned and your actual position. From an ephemeris you can find out where in the sky each astrologically important body was located, in relationship to the time and place you are considering.

Once you have selected a time and a location for astrological study and have gotten your cosmological information from the ephemeris, it is time to make up your horoscope.

HOROSCOPES: THE ROAD MAPS OF THE UNIVERSE

A horoscope is a *geocentric* map (one that assumes that the Earth is the center of the solar system) that records the *apparent* position of the sun and the moon and various stars and planets at any given moment of time. That time can be in the past, present, or future.

To form this map, draw a circle and divide it into 12 equal sections. These sections of the circle represent different sections of the sky. They are called

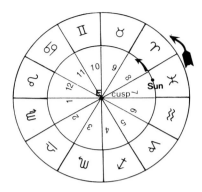

houses. This name comes from the astrological idea that we dwell in or under the physical and spiritual effects of the cosmos. Each house is different from the others because it represents a different section of the sky. And each section of the sky contains its own, ever-changing array of stars, constellations, and planets. Each house is related to one of the 12 astrological constellations. These are the *zodiac signs.*

The houses, or the 12 sections of the horoscope map, are each identified with one constellation, one planet, and a set of general human characteristics. The influences attributed to any planet or sign that enters any house is always evaluated as it relates to and reacts with the inherent nature of the house. That nature has been determined by the general nature of the sun sign that is related to it and by a long history of observation of human nature.

It is believed, by the way, that when the 12-house astrological chart was first devised the constellations identified with each house actually were located in that specific portion of the sky. Today, that has changed. Because of a phenomenon called the procession of the equinox, the elliptical nature of the planets' orbits, and the optical illusions caused by the motion of stars on different planes, the constellations shift their apparent positions slowly, year after year. A complete cycle of the procession of the equinox takes 25,800 years.

The following are the characteristics of each house:

First House: An individual's life, self, and general potentials. Related sign: Aries. Related Planet: Mars.

Second House: An individual's possessions and money. Related sign: Taurus. Related planet: Venus.

Third House: An individual's education and peer-group connections. Related sign: Gemini. Related planet: Mercury.

Fourth House: An individual's residence and relationship to parent of opposite sex. Related sign: Cancer. Related planet: Moon.

Fifth House: An individual's love relationships and children. Related sign: Leo. Related planet: Sun.

Sixth House: An individual's work and health. Related sign: Virgo. Related planet: Mercury.

Seventh House: An individual's partnerships, including spouse. Related sign: Libra. Related planet: Venus.

Eighth House: An individual's death or inheritance. Related sign: Scorpio. Related planet: Mars.

Ninth House: An individual's spiritual and intellectual life. Related sign: Sagittarius. Related planet: Jupiter.

Tenth House: An individual's career, repute, and social standing. Related sign: Capricorn. Related planet: Saturn.

Eleventh House: An individual's friendships and goals. Related sign: Aquarius. Related planet: Uranus.

Twelfth House: An individual's illness and troubles. Related sign: Pisces. Related planet: Neptune.

On a horoscope "map" the houses remain constant; the sun and the planets and constellations are assumed to pass through them. Do not be confused by the fact that a constellation is sometimes positioned in a house which is named for another constellation. For example, Pisces moves across the sky and consequently through our chart, entering each house including the 12th, with which it is related.

116

CHARTING YOUR HOROSCOPE

There are two basic types of horoscopes: 1. a natal horoscope (of your birth), and 2. a life horoscope (of any day, month or year).

A natal horoscope determines, in great detail, the location in the sky of all the planets, sun, moon, asteroids, and constellations, at the exact minute of your birth, in relation to the exact location of your birth.

A life horoscope considers the effect of the positions of the sun, moon, planets, asteroids, and constellations for any given day in your life, on some event in your life, past, present, or future.

Whichever horoscope you have charted, there are certain pieces of information that must be recorded on the horoscope. The sun, the moon, the planets, asteroids, and constellations must be positioned in the appropriate houses, depending on where they were in relationship to you at the time you are considering. The most important information is the location of your sun, moon, and rising and descending signs. They are explained below.

THE KEY PARTS OF A HOROSCOPE

The sun sign. The most influential single component of anyone's astrological horoscope is the sun sign. Your sun sign is basically determined by the location of the sun in the sky at your time of birth. This means that if you were born in July, the sun appears to be in that portion of the sky represented on a horoscope as the second house, Taurus. Therefore, your sun sign would be Taurus.

Bear in mind that astrology, an ancient and primitive science, still operates on the assumption that the sun revolves around the earth. This accounts for the fact that the sun sign is determined by the "changing position of the sun," a premise that is no longer scientifically sound, but which conforms to the appearance of reality.

The sun's power. As the sun is the energy source for our solar system, so is it the energy source for each person. Astrologically, the sun is the cosmic body that gives us vitality, power, and self-expression. How that drive is manifested in each of us individually is tempered by the position of the sun in the sky at the time of our birth.

The moon sign. The moon, which travels in a fast, repetitive cycle around the earth every 28 days, has long been thought to exert mysterious influence over us. Such physically observable facts as the moon's influence on the tides, the lunar-related cycle of menstruation, and moon-activated responses in sea creatures, have confirmed this supposition. These fluctuations—in response to the moon—have led astrologers to equate the moon's influence over human behavior with passion and changeability. It is no coincidence that our language uses words like lunacy, moon-struck, and going through a phase to describe unconscious erratic behavior.

The moon is placed on our natal chart to help us determine the nature of our intuitive and unconscious drives.

Rising signs: ascendants and descendants. As we have mentioned already, a horoscope is determined by both time and place. Place is important because the horizon—our range of sight—changes as we move north and south on the face of the Earth. We cannot see those heavenly bodies that are hidden from our view by the curve of the Earth.

Picture a circle. Choose a point on its surface. Draw a line tangent to the circle through that point. You will have described a horizon for that point. Now, if that point is Chicago and you are standing on the shores of Lake Michigan, it means that you will be able to see the part of the sky that is above that line. As the Earth revolves daily on its axis, it appears that the stars in the sky are passing above us. The Earth's motion from east to west makes different constellations appear at the furthest corner of our vision. Orion may appear low in the eastern sky at nine o'clock some winter night, but by midnight it will be directly above us. Many other stars will have risen above the horizon in those 3 hours.

Our rising sign is determined by finding out what constellation was appearing on our horizon at the minute of our birth. If we were born not in Chicago but, say, Fargo, South Dakota, on November 6, 1948 at 3:16 P.M., Pisces would have been the constellation that was rising on our horizon at that time. Someone born on the same day, at the same hospital, but 5 minutes later would have a different rising sign. For as the Earth's rotation is constant, so too is the rotation of rising signs.

Our descending sign is that constellation that was disappearing from our range of sight, dropping below our horizon line, at our time and place of birth.

Rising signs are thought to have an influence on both personality and physical appearance. Descendant signs are associated with our private or hidden aspects.

The planets. Besides the Earth, there are eight planets in our solar system: Mercury, Venus, Mars, Jupiter, Saturn, Uranus, Neptune, and Pluto. There are also four tiny planets, known as asteroids, which are located between Mars and Jupiter. They are Ceres, Pallas, Juno, and Vesta. Each of these bodies moves in an elliptical orbit around the sun, at a known distance from the sun, and at a specific speed.

It is the positions of these planets in relationship to the location and time of our birth that we put into our horoscope map. Each planet is said to exert a general influence on human behavior. That is why we must consider our horoscope daily if we want to find out what planetary influences will be exerted on us from day to day. Bear in mind that although the city of New York— with its 10 million residents—has the same daily sky chart for each of those persons, the effect of that chart is different for each individual. This is because the influence of the daily sky is tempered and altered by each individual's natal chart. This means that a person who is a Libra, with Pisces rising, may respond aggressively to the presence of Mercury on a specific day. But a person governed by Cancer may not feel the effects so strongly. These refinements can become very well defined when all aspects of a natal chart are considered in relation to a daily sky chart.

The general influences of the planets (untempered by their relationship to any other astrological forces) are:

Mercury—communication
Venus—gratification
Mars—initiative and action
Jupiter—expansion
Saturn—contraction
Uranus—individuality

Neptune—dependency
Pluto—obsession
The asteroids—various aspects of the "feminine" nature

In addition to these general powers, the planets exert specific influences on our temperaments and physical self when considered in relation to our sun sign and to each other.

REFINING YOUR HOROSCOPE

In order to make your horoscope appropriate to *you*, astrologers have subdivided the sun signs (Pisces, Aries, etc.) into specific groups that are said to govern particular temperamental qualities. These subdivisions are called the triplicities and the quadruplicities.

The triplicities are four groups of three sun signs. These groups are known as fire, air, earth, and water. Each group serves specific functions explained below:

1. *The Function of Fire: Feeling*
Aries, Leo, and Sagittarius are fire signs. The fire-ruled signs are said to possess the ability to project themselves and command attention. Usually, an individual born under a fire sign displays leadership ability.

Aries is enthusiastic, courageous, spearheads new efforts, likes to be first in doing something.

Leo is an actor or the central figure within a group; this sun sign craves attention.

Sagittarius is captivating, capable of becoming a philosophical or spiritual leader.

2. *The Function of the Earth: Practicality*
Taurus, Virgo, and Capricorn are earth signs. The earth-ruled signs are said to deal with reality. Usually, an individual born under an earth sign displays a skill for using and managing material resources.

Taurus is a sensualist who responds to things around him; he is concerned with value and money.

Virgo deals with work and service and is connected to health and healing.

Capricorn has the ability to structure things, be they the makings of a business empire or a coat.

3. *The Function of Air: Mental Ability*
Gemini, Libra, and Aquarius are air signs. The air-ruled signs deal with intellectual abilities, including communication and the capacity for forming social relationships. Usually, an individual born under an air sign evinces social and intellectual qualities.

Gemini displays curiosity and is anxious to share any observations made.

Libra reflects the ability to give attention to another person and can balance information and make comparisons.

Aquarius represents scientific, theoretical thinking and a concern for man's universal well-being.

4. *The Function of Water: Sensitivity*
Cancer, Scorpio, and Pisces are water signs. The water-ruled signs deal with

intuition, emotion, and feelings about life's deeper, psychic aspects. Usually, an individual born under a water sign displays perception and intuition.

Cancer represents strong feelings about home and family and is said to be the sign of a prophet.

Scorpio sees through pretense and facade and can be intense, even obsessive, and very creative.

Pisces possesses true empathy and can feel for others and, in an extreme form, live and respond through others.

The quadruplicities are three groups of four sun signs—each group connected with a quality that governs our general attitude to life and the way that we interrelate with people. The four general attitudes are explained below.

1. *Cardinal* Signs—extroverts concerned with the moment and present activities

2. *Fixed* Signs—introverts, concerned with the future and ideals

3. *Mutable* Signs—people who like to be part of a group, concerned with the past.

The order of the signs of the zodiac determines which signs belong to which quadruplicity. There are twelve signs of the zodiac. The year is divided into four seasons: spring, summer, fall, and winter. The first zodiac sign of each season—that is, Aries (spring), Cancer (summer), Libra (autumn), and Capricorn (winter)—is a Cardinal sign. The second zodiac sign of each season—Taurus (spring), Leo (summer) Scorpio (autumn), and Aquarius (winter)—is a Fixed sign. The last zodiac sign of each season—Gemini (spring), Virgo (summer), Sagittarius (autumn), and Pisces (winter) is a Mutable sign.

After these elements are plotted, further refinements are made to each chart. Relationships between the planets' positions is studied; the absence of certain planets on a chart can be as important as the presence of others. Every nuance is explored in an attempt to make the correlations between cosmic positions and personal events as individual and specific as possible.

DOES ASTROLOGY TELL FORTUNES?

When an astrologer looks at a horoscope calculated by a person's birth data, the relationships between the many factors mentioned above are all taken into consideration. And, as we have seen, every person is an astrological recipe made up of many differing ingredients. Given all this information, then, what precisely can astrology reveal to individuals about their lives?

Respectable astrology *does not* attempt to tell fortunes. Some astrologers do go in for making superficial predictions—these are, essentially, what most popular horoscope columns offer. But serious theoreticians look askance at this practice.

How the signs, planets, houses, and zodiacal groupings of quadruplicities and triplicities grew to be endowed with specific definitions and properties is an outgrowth of thousands of years of astrologers' study of human behavior. Based on this body of knowledge, most astrologers maintain that astrology can explain an individual's potential for behavior and personality and foresee when tension, crisis, and points of decision-making *may* occur in a person's life.

After an astrologer casts a person's horoscope based on birth data, he can

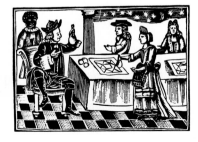

A seventeenth-century English cartoon shows an astrologer weighing bags of money taken from clients. In spite of scientific advances of the period, astrology remained popular with the majority of people.

then advance the chart to see how various components will be aligned at any given point in a person's lifetime.

At all times, cultural influences, of course, modify the strong tendencies that astrologers believe are an individual's legacy. For example, the planet Mercury, representing communication, might be prominent in two people's charts: Given the appropriate circumstances, one person might grow up to be the editor of a newspaper and the other might become a message carrier for a primitive tribe. How tendencies emerge or fail to emerge is the function of many variables having nothing to do with the astrological influences that exist in an individual's life.

Let us now look at the attributes and characteristics connected to each of the twelve sun signs of the zodiac, for as mentioned earlier, of all the components of a horoscope, the sun sign is by far the most significant.

THE ASTROLOGICAL TRAVELER

If you take your sun sign's information to heart, it could be interesting to go one step further and consider a vacation in astrological terms. If you're indecisive about what kind of vacation to plan, you might be helped by knowing that:

Aries, liking excitement, won't be happy with a ho-hum vacation, the same year in and year out. If she's scheduled to return to a past vacation site, she might vary her itinerary by including some bold new activities this trip—or choose a different exotic destination. Often a leader, an Aries traveler might be an ideal choice for a tour guide.

Taurus, who is thought to be concerned with value, will probably be most happy with a luxurious vacation. Or, on the other end of the spectrum, the value-conscious Taurus might be delighted with a bargain; an inexpensive cruise around the world on a tramp steamer might be just her speed.

Gemini, a people lover, is the born traveler. No matter where she roams, she's never alone for long. So she shouldn't be afraid to travel independently. Also to a Gemini's liking might be a stay at a lively hotel or resort filled with energetic people who keep going from morning until night.

Cancer likes her comfort and homelife. Separated from spouse or children, she might be lonely, so she'd be best off planning a family trip. Often a collector, a vacation might be the perfect time to start or expand a collection of beautiful things.

Leo, with a flair for the dramatic, would probably enjoy a stay at a snazzy hotel or ski resort, turning heads on the beach, slopes, or dance floor. Or, an African safari might appeal to the kingly lion or lioness. Wherever, a Leo's charm and vitality will heat up the immediate environment.

Virgo should resist her constant tendency to work and try to vacation in a luxurious location where, for a change, people will be waiting on her. But if this would make her feel guilty, she might plan a camping trip, which would both utilize her tremendous energy for working and ability to be at home in an outdoor setting.

Libra, with a tendency toward extremes, might like either an if-it's-Tuesday-it-must-be-Belgium tour or a solitary stay in a private villa. Perhaps the best vacation for a Libra would be one which had a little of each.

Scorpio rarely takes advice, so she might be better off planning her own vacation—no matter the hassles—than risk the possible annoyance of working with an agent who might not be sensitive to her needs. With her flair for problem-solving and dependable creativity, a no-itinerary vacation could turn out to be an exciting experience.

Sagittarius is often a sports enthusiast, so a rugged vacation—say, two weeks of sailing or scuba diving—might be more enjoyable than anything tame. This sun sign's amiability would make this traveler a welcomed member of a crew or team.

Capricorn, an unflagging worker who rarely shuns responsibility, needs a quiet vacation to compensate for the unrelenting pace that is her norm. Ruggedly independent, she would do well to get away from it all on a secluded island or mountaintop.

Aquarius, often a loner, might feel trapped by crowded restaurants, inns, or planes. So traveling off-season would make sense for this sun sign's optimally pleasant vacation. A quiet place where she could think in peace would be ideal.

Pisces, liking people as she does, would benefit from contact with others. Give her a friendly chalet, where she can ski by day and sip wine by the fireside at night. Such a romantic setting would appeal to her highly emotional nature.

10. Planning a Sunny Vacation

Whether you plan to chase the sun from continent to continent or spread your beach towel on the closest sandy shore, you'll want to do everything you can before you leave home to make sure that you will have a truly carefree, relaxing sojourn.

To help with all your big plans (and little odds and ends) this chapter takes you through each step of planning a vacation in the sun: There are questions to help you determine what you *really* want out of your vacation; tips on selecting and working with a travel agent; valuable pointers on packing, choosing luggage, and planning for special activities—all designed to help you take care of the business of travel, and get on to the fun.

ANALYZING YOUR ATTITUDE

We don't need years with a psychiatrist to know that when we bathe in a cool inlet by late-day sun, our troubles—momentarily, at least—seem to float away with every lapping wave. But a trip to the sun can be more than a temporary release from stress or the blahs. A sun vacation can respond to a great many of our needs, if we take them into account when we plan our trip. The key is to get to know your travel temperament. Ask yourself the following questions. Your answers will help you realize what you want, need, expect, and can actually anticipate from your sun adventure.

What are the main goals of your trip? Sleep? A tan? Meeting people? Seeing sights? Culture? Nightlife? Sports?

What style vacation do you want? Formal or barefoot? Subdued or flamboyant? Simple or elegant? Social or solitary?

What do you think you will gain from your trip? A new lease on life? A chance to unwind? A reasonable interlude from familiar surroundings? Educational experience? Sorely missed excitement? Opportunity to indulge a special interest or activity? A cure for a broken heart?

With the answers to these questions in mind you can begin a vacation that suits you, tailoring it to your needs and tastes. You will also be able to see whether your expectations are realistic, and if they can be fulfilled, given proper planning.

SELECTING AND USING TRAVEL AGENTS

Now you have a good idea of what you want, but where in the world are you going to find it? How to begin? Where to go for advice?

Self-help is, of course, one of today's buzzwords; there are indeed those among us who feel compelled to do for ourselves. We grow our own vegetables, teach ourselves Italian or English, and repair automobiles. But plan a vacation? *This* is truly a job for an expert.

The sun, the sand, and the silk smooth waves greet sun worshippers at Bermuda's Mid-ocean Beach.

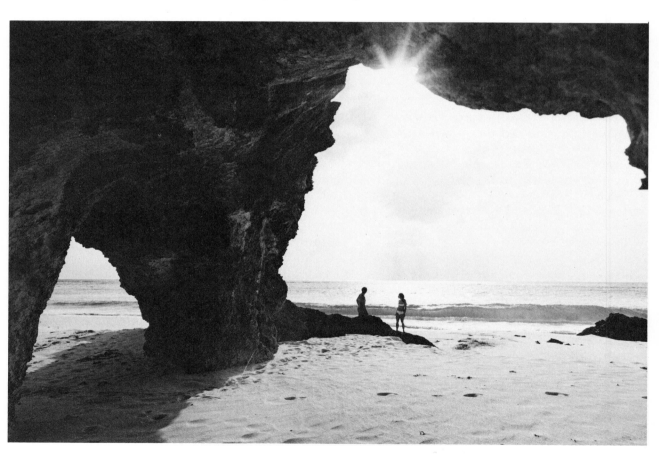

WORKING WITH THE TRAVEL AGENT

When you've found an agent with whom you feel comfortable, the first service they can offer you is advice: How much should you expect your trip to cost? What is the best hotel or resort for you? What should you leave out of your itinerary? However, an agent can only help *you* when you help *them*. In order to get the best guidance, your agent should know specifically what you like and need. Outline your lifestyle: What kind of food do you enjoy? What activities are your favorites? Do you prefer quiet or excitement? Are you a day person or a night person? What luxuries are your necessities? How much money are you willing to spend? Do you like music? Dance? Art? Architecture? Archaeology? Sports? Let your agent know *why* you are planning your trip and *how* you want to travel.

A WORD ON CHOOSING CRUISING

Don't overlook cruises. Although their reputation has taken a turn for the tacky, there are still ships with glamour and charm intact. Besides, for pure relaxation, leisure time at sea can often beat the relative hustle and bustle of land vacationing. After all, you need never hail a taxi.

When choosing a cruise, avoid anything billed for swinging singles or so long a trip that it is bound to attract only the idle, boring, and ancient. Look for ships with casual atmosphere and open rooms that encourage mingling. Again, with specialty cruises a recent trend, following one's own interest, be it scuba diving or studying the occult, can lead to the best results.

PACKING FOR THE SUN

Once you've planned your trip, your next assignment is finding a way of bringing your possessions (and the right ones) along with you to the sun. It's a delicate matter, packing. On the one hand, you don't want to be burdened like a packhorse and risk suffering terminal muscle ache as you drag a burgeoning bag. But then, why spoil a trip by showing up without a bathing suit in, say, Antigua, only to learn that it has a different beach for every day of the year (yes, 365).

The trick in packing is to travel as lightly as possible, but with all the gear you'll need to make your trip a smash. The first thing you must consider is how large and heavy your luggage can be and still be allowed on a commercial flight. Oceanliners permit transatlantic passengers to bring 8 pieces of stateroom luggage and 2 small trunks (no larger than 30 cubic feet per trunk). Excess baggage costs $2 per cubic foot—minimum $10. Cruise passengers are limited to 2 standard-sized suitcases.

Free baggage allowance regulations on commercial airplanes are both confusing and rather arbitrarily enforced:

Within the U.S., both in coach and first-class sections, you may *carry on* luggage if its total measurements—determined by adding its height plus length plus width—do not exceed 45 inches. You may *check* two bags—one no larger than 62 inches, the other no larger than 55 inches (determined by the same formula), and each weighing less than 70 pounds.

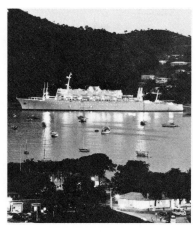

Cruise ships add a festive glow to the evening landscape at Charlotte Amalie in St. Thomas.

125

On international flights, planes departing the U.S. allow first-class passengers a *carry on* piece no more than 45 inches overall and two *checked* pieces measuring no more than 62 inches each.

Coach passengers may *carry on* a bag 45 inches overall and may *check* 2 bags that total 106 inches (with no one bag larger than 68 inches).

It is a sensible precaution to weigh your bags at home before departure. Because even though they are not weighed in at the time you leave the U.S.—chances are that upon returning to the U.S. from a foreign airport your bags will be weighed.*

Selecting luggage. Your second packing step is to take a critical look at the luggage you own, to see if you have, in fact, one or more pieces appropriate to your needs. If you're still carrying the hard-sided luggage that your parents bought you when you graduated from school fifteen years ago, it might be time to shop for something lighter, more practical. Or if all you have is a giant Valpak—fine for your husband's suits but entirely wrong for weekend ski gear—you'd be infinitely better off borrowing or purchasing a smaller bag, right for weekending.

There are two basic categories of luggage: carry-on bags and larger suitcases. You will want to consider what style bag will serve you best in both categories.

For larger suitcase bags, weight is a major consideration. You cannot depend on a doorman or skycap to be available when you need them. And lugging luggage gives real meaning to the word!

Look into softsided luggage. Usually, it's lightweight. (Not always, though, particularly if you favor sumptuous but sturdy leather.) Besides their generally lighter weight, softsided bags have the advantages of being easy to carry, expandable (there always seems to be room to squeeze in one last black-pearl necklace from Tahiti or even a native Jamaican basket), and kind to clothing.

Canvas is generally a good choice of material for softsided luggage. But these days you should shop around. Look into parachute silk, nylon, even some straws. And if weight or price isn't so important to you, a beautifully tanned cowhide or buttery Italian suede could still be your bag.

There are those who swear by the usual rectangular, hinged bags; others who say that a duffel is more workable. But like in most things, shape is largely a matter of taste. It's size that counts.

For short trips, carry-on luggage makes sense. Who, after all, wants to waste a precious half-hour waiting for one's grip to make a grand entrance?

Some people can squeeze all they need for a weekend into a compact 45 inches. Whether or not you're such a wizard, try to use luggage that is sensibly sized. When in doubt, take two smallish pieces; you will find them easier to manipulate than one enormous one.

In choosing carry-on luggage, look for a style that offers several separate compartments, including one zippered, outside section. This spot is the ideal place for things you may need to get at in a hurry—your plane ticket, perhaps, or hotel confirmation.

---

*This is because many foreign countries still use old weight-determined baggage allowance rules. The U.S. size regulations are new. Therefore, an unfortunate traveler risks being levied an overweight charge on the identical bags, which were, only a week before, given the U.S. stamp of approval based on their overall size!

What to pack. Your third step is filling your bags. What to take is a highly personal problem, but there are basic rules of thumb that can help make your sun vacation go smoothly.

Do research. Ask your friends and travel agent, check the fashion pages of magazines and newspapers. The point is to discover what people are wearing *now.* Even if you've visited a place before, many spots have become more informal. For evening, a few bare dresses might do where before you'd feel compelled to wear a stiff ensemble. In many locations—if you have the lean body for them—a sexy pair of jeans can see you through almost any outing.

Pack for the right climate, weather, and temperature. If you'll be touring in hot weather, remember to bring light, loose-fitting skirts or pants, and don't forget that where there's heat, there's often air-conditioning; a shawl, light linen blazer, or sweater is a must. Remember that not only clothing, but also cosmetics must be varied to suit the climate. Dry heat or bitter cold may require a richer moisturizer and lip balm. In high humidity you may feel the need for a water, not oil, based foundation, or a refreshing facial mask.

Concentrate on comfort. The uppercrust of Abidjan may dress to the nines. It doesn't mean you have to, as long as you're decently clad.

Bali's street vendors can supply an over-packed traveler with handy woven totes.

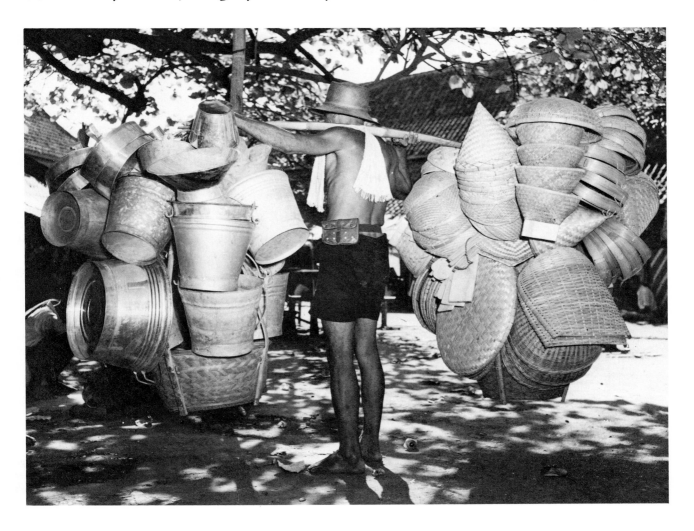

When you select clothing, consider what will look well on you when you're tanned.

Pack only what you're certain you'll wear—comfy ski clothing, flattering tops, a knockout beach coverup—and leave behind marginal items you *think* you should wear. If something's too tight, doesn't go with other things you're bringing, or takes up half your suitcase, leave it at home.

Don't bring anything new that you haven't tried on or gotten used to.

Aim for a basic color scheme. But don't lock yourself in to the point where you tire so of your vacation wardrobe you want to donate it to charity.

Look for clothing that works well in both day and evening.

Bring as few accessories as possible, bearing in mind the rule above. They tend to weigh the most and get worn the least.

Pick items which resist wrinkling and are easy to maintain. Of course, many man-made fibers have this distinction. But don't kiss off all natural ones. Crinky Indian cotton, gauzy silk noil, and many other real fabrics may be less perishable than you imagine.

Pick the garment of better quality, when choosing between two garments. It will probably look fresher longer.

Bring local currency. Check with your agent to find the easiest method of getting some foreign currency with which to begin your trip. Usually, major banks offer this service.

Keep a list of your passport number, traveler's check numbers, and credit card numbers; tuck it away safely apart from the carry-on bag or handbag that houses these valuables.

Special note: Never check through valuable documents, medicine, tickets, traveler's checks, manuscripts, eye glasses, contact lenses, or contraceptives. These items should be packed in your carry-on bag along with practical things you may need enroute, such as makeup, sunglasses, reading material, foreign phrase book, or slippers. It is a good idea to also bring along an extra prescription for medications and eye glasses or contact lenses, a list of doctors recommended by your physician at home, and list of important health information—medications you take, allergies, blood type, names and addresses of your doctors.

TAKE-OUT FOR THE SUN

Whether you're off to humid tropics or arid deserts, to the Alps or the frozen fjords you will want to pack toiletries, cosmetics, skin- and hair-care products that will protect your skin, enhance your tan, add shine to your hair and a healthy glow to your face. Although certain types of basic toiletries, such as toothpastes or first aid creams, are readily available the world over—you cannot depend on your favorite cosmetic or the best sun lotions to be available at your local palm tree, so be sure the following find a place in your bags:

Sun protection lotions. Suntan lotion, sun screens, sun blocks, or sun enhancers—whatever you need and want. These are important because foreign brands are often expensive and do not all rate their effectiveness according to the Sun Protection Factor System (SPF).

Skin moisturizers. Water, wind, sun, and snow can chafe and parch your skin, making it susceptible to wrinkling, chapping and peeling.

Lip balms. Particularly necessary to protect your lips from burning and cracking.

Light beach wraps, easy to pack, can make your swimwear exotic and beautiful.

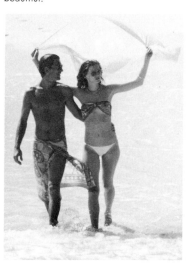

128

Sun-screening makeup. For extra sun protection check labels to see if special ingredients are in the makeup.

Cooling skin fresheners. For hot weather sunning, apply to your wrists, temples, back of your knees, to cool you off and add a gentle scent.

Hair care products. Antidryness shampoos, conditioners, and rinses soothe your battered hair. Sun, wind, and water can dry and damage your tresses. Combs, pins, and barrettes help control wet and wind-blown hair.

Sunburn soothers. If you misjudge your sun endurance you'll need a soothing—perhaps minty—lotion, thick enough to really adhere to your skin and keep it from losing any more moisture.

PHOTOGRAPHING IN THE SUN

We live in a world of instant images, elaborate cameras, and fanatic shutter-bugs; no place on earth is free of the inquiring eye of the amateur (and professional) photographer. We have all come to depend on the chronicle that our camera produces, for our vacation memories are formed as much by our pictures as by our own, often untrustworthy recall. Good photos, properly exposed and properly composed, are simply a matter of following a few guidelines and knowing the trick of photographing under the special conditions found in the sun.

Selecting your subjects. You will want to take all those standard—but nice—photos of friends and relations, hotels, and cabanas that you have seen. "Me and the kids at the Eiffel Tower." "Gladys and Fred in the boat." But you may also want to capture something of the feeling of your sun spot—the smell of its flora, the soft caress of its ocean breezes, the texture of its landscape—or you can direct your attention to the flowers, birds, shells, and even fish that surround you. Each type of subject requires a different photographic approach. Small objects must be dealt with differently than groups of people. The shade produces different photographic problems than full sun. The following tips can help you get the best results from your camera—in any sun situation.

When you are photographing people, remember:

• Choose a simple background, which will not compete with the subjects of your photo.

• If standing, subjects should hold themselves erect, place one leg slightly in front of the other, and stretch tall. This achieves a slender look.

• Straight-on poses are usually the least flattering. Subject should turn slightly away from the camera.

• In photos where the subject is seated, she should avoid slouching. Legs should be crossed at the ankles rather than knees.

• A thin person's figure will look fuller if she is seated.

• A one-piece suit, cut high on the leg, is more flattering in photos than a bikini.

• Sunglasses should be removed.

• A partial torso view, taken from the waist up, can be a good alternative to a full body view.

If you decide to take close-up pictures of small objects such as shells, flowers, or insects, Kodak suggests:

• Use a simple background. If a flower, for instance, can't be moved to a noncompeting background, place a piece of colored paper behind it, arranging the paper so that the flower doesn't cast a shadow.

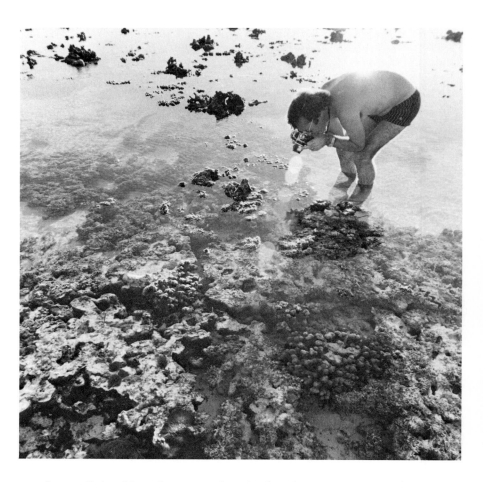

- In sun, light objects from the side or back. Sidelighting will emphasize shape through highlights and shadows. Backlighting will point up any translucency.
- Avoid patchy lighting; choose either total sun or shade.
- Consider taking pictures on overcast days; lighting then will be soft and even—good for photographing detail.
- Without a close-up lens, 4 to 5 feet is a good distance to put between your camera and a small object.

You may find yourself coping with special problems.
- Protect your camera from direct sunlight, especially if the temperature exceeds 110 degrees, which may easily happen when a camera is kept in a glove compartment or left on a sunny beach. Store your camera in a leather case and shady place, such as your picnic basket (which you can keep cool with a moistened towel) or in an air-conditioned car. Remember to give camera and film time to warm up to a higher temperature when you use them.
- Humidity can harm film, causing color to appear washed out and causing black-and-white to look murky. In climates with humidity above 65 percent, keep film dry by storing it in a refrigerator. Take it out a night before it is to be used, which will allow any condensation to evaporate. In tropical climates, humidity is its lowest during daytime, your best time to load a camera.

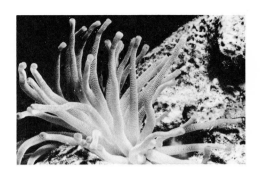

- Water can ruin film and rust camera parts. Protect film and camera from sea spray, mist, rain, snow, and perspiration. For example, in a boat, store a camera in a plastic case or bag.
- Sand and dust can scratch a lens or penetrate tiny crevices. At the beach, use a clear filter over your lens. If sand or dust find their way inside a camera, blow them out.
- In cold, allow warm equipment to cool to nature's temperature before removing from cases in order to minimize condensation, which can cause icing.
- To avoid frostbite, a cold-weather photographer should wear a thin pair of gloves under heavier gloves and keep the thin pair on when he uses his camera.
- Snow reflection can cause overexposure. To judge light accurately, a meter should be held close to a subject or the back of the photographer's hand.

Underwater photography for beginners. Snorkelers and scuba divers, even if novices, can bring back striking photographs with less trouble than they might expect with this advice from Kodak:
- Use a watertight plastic camera housing, available through camera or scuba shops.
- Many cameras are adaptable to underwater picture-taking. To be sure yours will do, check it with professionals at your local camera or scuba shops.
- Water absorbs, blocks, and scatters light. Close to the surface, where the light is brightest, you'll have the best chance of taking clear shots. In deeper water, the color will be less intense. For maximum light, take pictures that are front-lighted. (This means: the sun is coming over your shoulders.)
- To attract fish, offer them chum-bread or fish food—they will gobble it up while you shoot.
- In or out of the water, you want to be steady when you take pictures. If you can't brace yourself by holding a stationary object, stand or kneel. If swimming toward a subject, move slowly.
- A wide-angle lens can help compensate for mistakes in aim.

SANDCASTLES

Sandcastle building is not child's play. You must have the imagination of an artist and the nerves of a tightrope walker. For a true castle builder creates an image of her royal aspirations—right at the crestline of high tide. There is no doubt that the waves will wash your palace away, but for a few hours before the tide turns, you can make your fortress the ultimate place in the sun.

To build your castle, you will need:

a large bucket in which to mix sand and water;

a small pail or cup for transporting water from the sea to your territory;

a spatula for scooping out and flattening down a large area;

a sharp knife for cutting out details, such as windows and turrets;

a thin piece of metal wire for cutting deep into interior sections of walls and mounds;

interestingly shaped pieces of wood, metal, etc., for making forms, designs, and molding curves and archways; and

a flat, solid wood block (or blocks of various sizes) for tamping down wet sand.

Once you have assembled these things, you can begin construction.

The most important part of any sand castle is the foundation. If you have a weak base, one that cracks or crumbles, you will jeopardize whatever you build.

First, draw a circle in the sand about 10 feet in diameter. Sprinkle a bucket of water over the sand so it is moist but not soaked. Pat down all the sand very firmly so it is solid and even. Sprinkle with more water.

Bring in more sand from outlying areas and heap it the middle of the circle. Spread the sand out so that it is thicker in the middle than around the edges. Sprinkle with water and pat down firmly.

Bring in more sand, sprinkle with water, and pat. Repeat this process until you have constructed a cone-shaped mound about 2 feet high in the center and one foot high on the edges.

There should be no dry spots, no air bubbles, and no crumbling sand.

Now you are ready to *form the basic shape.*

Fill your bucket half full of sand. Add water and mix until you have a thick cement like goo. Not runny—solid, but wet.

Begin to make thick rough walls and thin tall mounds—for turrets and spires. Pack everything firmly so no air bubbles will make it crack as it dries.

Add roadways, general shapes for other buildings, a moat, and other large details. Take your time with this step. Get a good rough shape, with all the parts and forms you want. Don't detail anything until everything is done roughly. Keep your sand and water mixture thick. Pat everything firmly.

Now you are ready for the hard part—the details: arches, spires, doors, windows, cannons, gardens (hanging and otherwise), etc.

Start at the top. Once you have established the basic shape, you should work from the top down. Spires, turrets, ramparts, etc., are the first objects that deserve your attention, so that if they crumble and fall they will not damage anything below them. Don't make the spires and towers too steep—be slightly humble.

Use reinforcements for all bridges, overpasses, and arches—sticks, shells, wire, anything to strengthen the structure. Try wood-centered columns where strength is of optimum importance.

There are those who feel that moats should be filled with water, and there are those who feel that moats should remain empty until the encroaching tide fills them. An empty moat will help preserve the castle for a few more minutes —another attempt to stave off the inevitable forces of decay. It is a philosophic decision.

II. On the Beach

This section is devoted to those special creatures, natives to the world's sun spots, that greet us when we arrive. On the land (and sometimes at sea) butterflies trace colorful, graceful patterns in the air. At our feet, flowers crowd toward the beaches and sprinkle themselves across mountain meadows, straining toward the sun, knowing well how lovely life in the sun can be. At the shoreline we find shells of myriad shapes and sizes tantalizing us with the mystery and complexity of life under water. And fish—glorious and bizarre quarry for snorkelers and divers—fill the sea with colors and shapes far more exotic than we might ever imagine. What follows is a sampling of the creatures and curiosities of the sunbelt.

BUTTERFLIES

What is a butterfly? Believe it or not, it is an insect that evolves from a cocoon, lives a brief seasonal life, helps pollinate plants, causes few problems, and delights everyone. There are thousands and thousands of different types. Brazil alone is known to have more than 600 different species. These flightly beauties travel—some migrate several thousand miles each season—and are seen a thousand miles out to sea relentlessly beating their wings, heading for their summer sun spot. Passengers on cruise ships often find a lone butterfly resting upon a deck railing or a swarm of butterflies following their boat's southbound route.

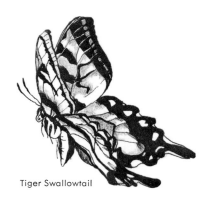

Tiger Swallowtail

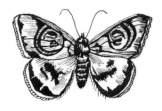

African Cyligramma

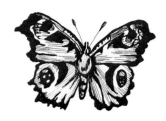

Peacock

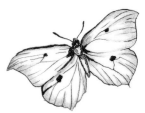

Asian Brimstone

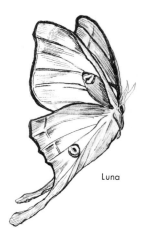

Luna

The TIGER SWALLOWTAIL is a common North American species. You can see it dressed in long formal tails of orange, yellow, and black in grassy meadows and coastal wetlands. Its European cousin is a more subtly colored version—somewhat smaller, but still resplendent.

The AFRICAN CYLIGRAMMA lives high among the tree tops of the forest where it munches on leaves and basks in the warm sunshine. It develops vivid coloring slowly after emerging from the cocoon.

The PEACOCK butterfly is one of 5000 similar species that are found throughout temperate and tropical areas. This butterfly flutters by on blue and green wings.

The ASIAN BRIMSTONE, pale green and flecked with red, graces the meadows and fields of Southeast Asia and China.

The LUNA is a spectacular moth that grows up to 3 inches in length—with an even larger wing span. Its pale wings and long swooping tails make it a candidate for the most beautiful insect in North America.

134

FLORA

Sun near a bank of wild Hawaiian ORCHIDS; ski past fields of EDELWEISS; smell the fragrance of Indian JASMINE; and sidestep the sticky grasping jaws of the tropics' VENUS FLYTRAP. Soothe your sunburn with the cool magic of the ALOE LILY, and warm your snow-chilled toes in a tea brewed of wild mountain clover. Treat your nose and your eyes to their beauty, for flowers are never far away from the world's best sun spots.

Collecting Wild Flowers. Throughout history flowers have been important to the world's great travelers. Marco Polo, Goethe, Columbus, Darwin, all investigated the vegetation as they traveled through new lands. They brought back specimens, living and dried, that changed their societies' concepts of the world's wonders.

In some areas today it is prohibited to pick flowers and other flora. *Always check* with your hotel clerk, tour guide, or local authorities before you set out to collect samples. If it is legal, be judicious. Don't take flowers you won't press and save.

If you are going to press flowers, the following equipment will be helpful:

Scissors or sharp razor. Don't tear the stem, you can damage the remaining plant and hurt your specimen, too.

Wax paper. This is best because it is heavy, moisture-resistant and nonreactive. Foils and plastics will stick and damage the flower.

One very heavy book. This is the press. Other flat heavy objects will do—but nothing ever works quite so well as an unabridged dictionary, or a Russian novel.

Note: If you are on an extended walk and you think your flowers might wilt before you get them back to your room, bring along a plastic bag filled with wet napkins or tissues. Put the stems of the flowers into this bag. This will help them retain their bright colors and firm shape until you press them.

These seven steps will guarantee beautiful results.

1. Choose fresh, unwilted specimens.

2. Pick with leaves and stem to show the whole plant structure.

3. Cut two sheets of waxed paper the size of your pressing book. Place one sheet on a page of an open book.

4. Place the specimen on the sheet. Place the leaves on the stem at a natural angle to the stalk. Lay them flat.

5. To press the flower, you may leave the petals up, covering the stamen, with front and back petals touching, or open flower so that petals form a circle around the center. The method of presentation you select should depend on the sturdiness of your flower. The hardy varieties can be pressed open.

6. Place a second piece of waxed paper over flower.

7. Close the book quickly. Weigh down the cover if needed.

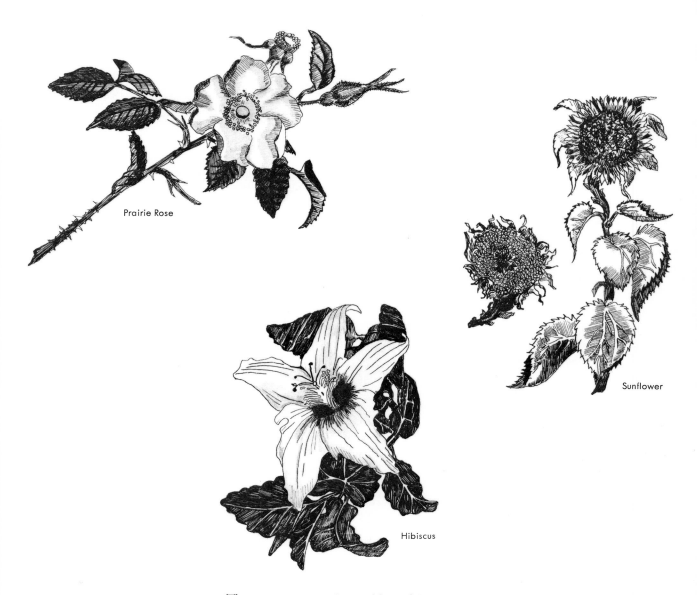

Prairie Rose

Sunflower

Hibiscus

The PRAIRIE ROSE is a wild rambling rose, common to the United States from Texas to New York, which blossoms from May to July, after which the rose hips (seed pods below blooms) may be picked for use as a tea.

From Oceania comes this huge 6-inch HIBISCUS flower. The petals are pink, white, and crimson, and the plant itself can grow up to 7 feet high.

SUNFLOWERS are a common wild flower and can be as small and delicate as a tiny daisy and as gargantuan as a sapling. Our common image is of the cultivated variety that grows up to 15 feet or more and has a single blossom that is 8 inches or more in diameter. Sunflower seeds are used for making oil and, when dried, can be eaten like nuts.

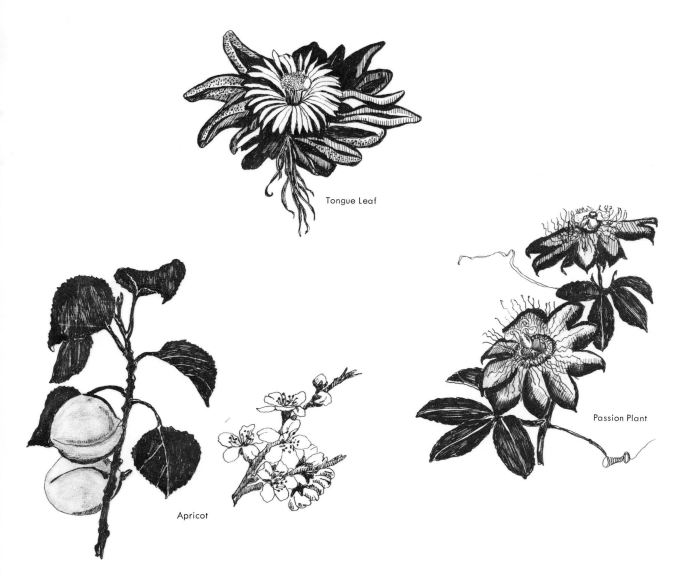

Tongue Leaf

Apricot

Passion Plant

A spring bloomer, the APRICOT is native to the Middle East. Cultivated else-where for their tasty fruit, they grow wild on the rough hillsides of Lebanon and Jordan.

The TONGUE LEAF is a ground-hugging plant that thrives in warm tropical climates. The scent of its large, handsome flower is said to have aphrodisiac powers.

PASSION PLANTS, also known as passion flowers, display their exotic blooms in the warm, humid tropics. Their unusual flower is crowned by a fringe of delicate filaments. European botanists thought the structure of the plant re-sembled the implements used in the Crucifixion—thus the name Passion Plant. The fruit is edible and is known as a Maypop.

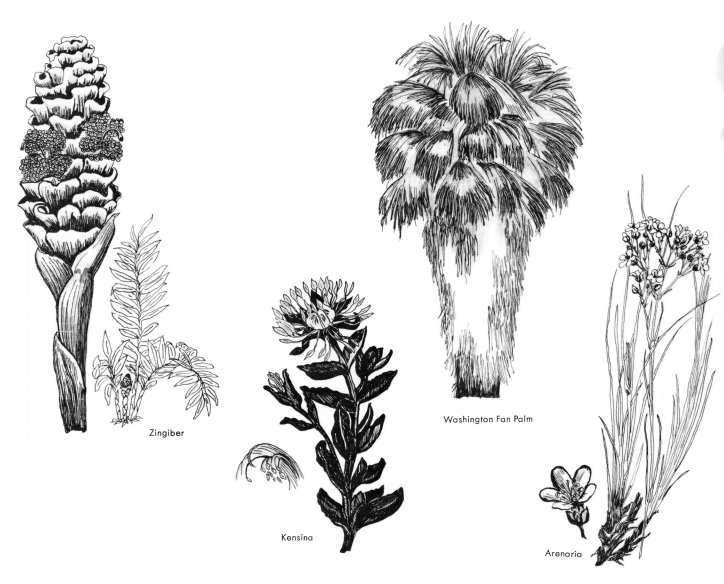

Zingiber

Kensina

Washington Fan Palm

Arenaria

Nine hundred exotic varieties of ZINGIBER are found throughout the tropics of the Eastern Hemisphere. Related to ginger, cardamom and turmeric, its flower is aromatic.

The KENSINA is crowned with a cluster of small spiked petals emanating from a brightly colored center. It is found in hot, humid climates.

Of the 14 varieties of palms native to the United States the WASHINGTON FAN PALM is the least well known and the most useful. Its fruit is an edible berry, a common food for Southwest Indians. Even today its fibrous tissue is used for brushes and brooms.

ARENARIA is a delicate wild flower with thin, wispy leaves and a long stem that is topped by a cluster of pale blooms one-quarter of an inch wide. Its many varieties are common in most temperate climates.

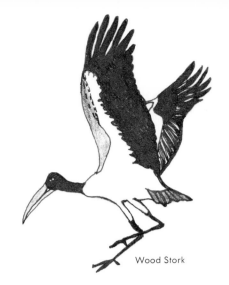

Wood Stork

BIRDS

"Birds gotta fly . . ." says the old song, but that lyric just "ain't necessarily so." Take the EMU or the OSTRICH, the KAGU and the KIWI, the PENGUIN and the flightless CORMORANT. These birds have small vestigial wings, some flappable, some not. But they couldn't get off the ground if their lives depended on it. (It doesn't, so they have survived.)

Many different types of birds inhabit almost all regions of the globe, from the Arctic Circle to the Amazon. They range from gentle chickadees to ferocious vultures. The one thing that many of these species have in common is the impulse to follow the sun. They have long-standing reservations at their favorite winter sun spots and often travel thousands of miles to get there. They are very loyal to their favorite resorts, and once there, they are reputed to live it up— eating well and donning bright plumage. These are the quintessential sun worshippers.

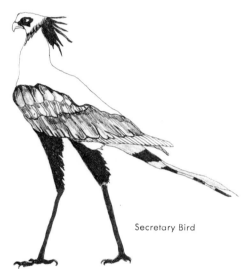

Secretary Bird

The WOOD STORK is a neighbor of the DARTER. It is found not only in Central and South America, but also in the inland waterways of Florida. In earlier eras, when America was more tropical, these birds were at home much farther north. But through the millennia, the American tropical zone has shrunk to a small area along the Gulf Coast and in Florida. As a consequence, these birds are isolated and vulnerable.

The SECRETARY BIRD, another long-legged species, strides across the sunny grasslands of western Africa. You wouldn't want this handsome creature along as a traveling secretary! They are strong-willed and strong-headed, and kick their adversaries to death! They are so named because the feathers that extend off the back of their heads reminded some colonial of the way secretaries looked with quill pens tucked behind their ears.

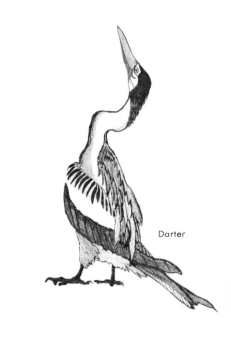

Darter

The DARTER, found in inland waters of Florida, swims with its entire body under water—only its long neck and head stick out above the surface. Its plumage is white and blue-gray. When out of the water, it has the habit of perching with its wings spread for long periods of time.

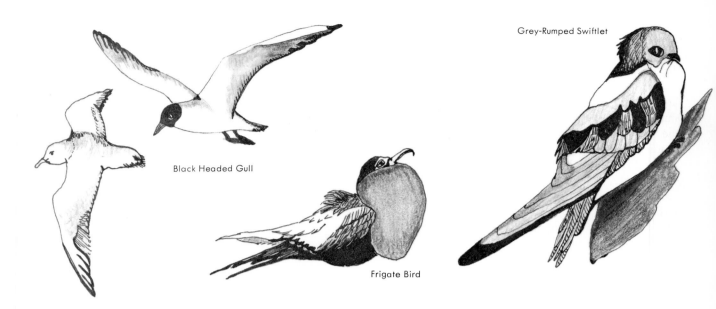

Grey-Rumped Swiftlet

Black Headed Gull

Frigate Bird

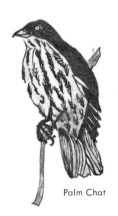

Palm Chat

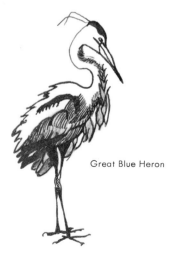

Great Blue Heron

Found from northern China to western France, the BLACK HEADED GULL is an habitué of inland waterways and coastal wetland alike. Like its cousins world wide it is an "opportunistic feeder" and will scavenge whatever it can—from fields and from the water.

The magnificent FRIGATE BIRD is another Caribbean marvel. This marauding, ill-mannered bird attacks other birds and steals food from them. The male, seen here, inflates his bright red neck sac to attract females. Once there are young birds in the nest, they must be constantly protected, for other Frigates will plunder the nest looking for building materials for their own home—and in the process kill the young ones.

Ever wonder about birds nest soup? Well, wonder no more. This GREY-RUMPED SWIFTLET is the source of this delicacy. Their "white nests" (the most prized variety) are made from thread-like filaments of their saliva. The Chinese have always claimed that these nests have not only special culinary virtues, but special medical ones as well. It is not an unreasonable claim, since the nests are composed of 50 percent protein and a high concentration of mineral salts.

The PALM CHAT lives only on the islands of Hispaniola and Gonave in the Caribbean. Very sociable birds, they are often found traveling in packs, exchanging thoughts with squeaks and buzzes—because they cannot sing! More extraordinary is the fact that they live in large apartment complexes about 10 feet high and 4 feet in diameter. They build these mounds out of interlaced twigs and as many as 30 couples share the space—each pair having their own private chamber.

This bony-legged water wader, the GREAT BLUE HERON, favors the inland waters of Florida, the Yucatan, and Cuba, where the crowds are thin and the sun is strong. Standing 4 feet tall, it is quite a sight, with its dark blue underfeathers, and blue and white neck plumage.

FISH

The 50 million or more years that have passed since life emerged from the seas has not erased love of the water from our basic human nature. Water is, literally, in our blood. But only fish (and a few shrewd mammals) have been smart enough to remain at home in the water, close to the great beaches of the world. We must travel many miles, deal with a great variety of plans and problems to get to the spots that fish call home.

The breathtaking variety of underwater life visible to the vacationing snorkeler is nothing short of dazzling. It makes the scuba divers' "rapture of the deep" perfectly understandable. Even fish that live far beneath the ocean's surface—away from sun, rarely seen by any man—display the most remarkable appearances, in color and design, of any of the world's creatures.

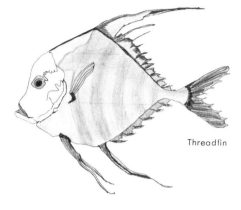

Threadfin

THREADFINS are an unusually large, flat fish. Sometimes they grow up to 5 feet, although smaller ones are more common. It is so named because of its thin, wispy fins, more pronounced on some varieties than on others. If you are visiting Maui or Micronesia, look for this funny face.

The big-eyed CARDINALFISH is a 4-inch showoff that likes to display its stripes and spots around the inlets and sunny shoals of Hong Kong and the Philippines.

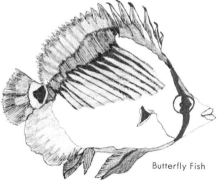

Cardinalfish

The BUTTERFLY FISH is another coral reef dweller seen throughout the Indian Ocean and the Pacific around Australia and New Zealand. A beautiful fish, pale bodied with golden fins and a wide black stripe on its face, it grows to about 7 inches. It is friendly, though somewhat shy—a much better fish to investigate than its neighbor the SPOTFIN.

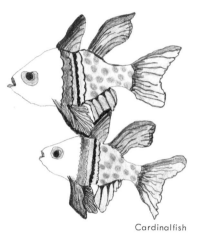

Butterfly Fish

Hooked, crooked, pugged, and pointed, there are no noses too unique for a fish. The green and yellow LONGNOSED FILEFISH is a prime example. A fast moving creature, it darts in and out of the shallow waters around reefs, poking into nooks and crannies, looking for tasty tidbits of young living coral.

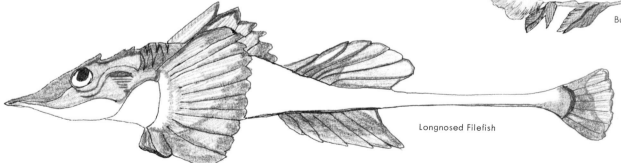

Longnosed Filefish

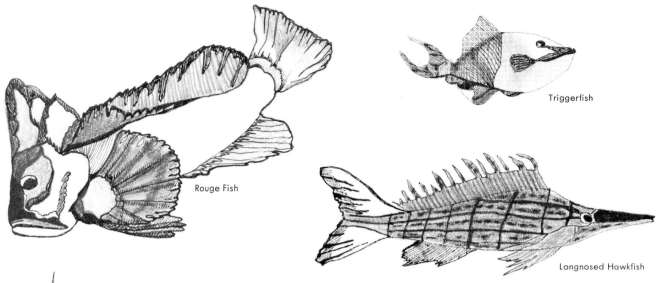

Triggerfish

Longnosed Hawkfish

Rouge Fish

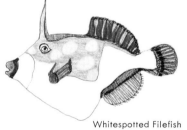

Whitespotted Filefish

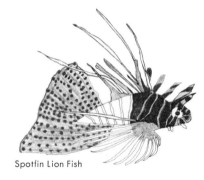

Spotfin Lion Fish

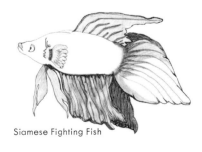

Siamese Fighting Fish

No need for blusher for this ROUGE FISH; it has its own natural glow—an orangey tint across its barnacled skin. A member of the unfriendly scorpion family, its dorsal fins contain a poison. So, when you are passing your time in the waters of Bali and Ceylon, beware this tiny 5-inch menace.

A local Caribbean resident, the TRIGGERFISH, has been seen as far north as Cape Cod. You will notice its slightly belligerent jaw line—the sharp teeth. It is small but tough, and other fish do well to avoid its teeth and its tail. We humans need not worry as long as we keep our fingers out of its mouth!

Another entrant in the Durante look-alike contest is the LONGNOSED HAWK-FISH. This splendid red and white plaid fish is a rarity and keeps to itself far beneath the surface (sometimes 100 feet deep!) in the waters around Baja and Hawaii.

What's blue and brown and spotted all over? A WHITESPOTTED FILEFISH of course. This rare fish—suspected of lifelong monogamy—gets bigger and bigger spots as it ages. Rarely seen, they dart in and out of the corals and underwater plants in the Caribbean.

Take, for example, the SPOTFIN LION FISH. This resident of the coral reefs in the China Sea and the South Pacific spends much of its time hanging upside down from the ceilings of dark coral grottoes, but it is not a dreary specimen. Its bright orange body, striped with white, and its brown and white fins are a vivid background for its long, poisonous spines. Although not an aggressive fish, it will strike out when provoked. So don't try to get too close!

The Oriental martial arts for fish? Well, it happens. SIAMESE FIGHTING FISH are a form of carp that have been developed through careful breeding and selection. They are unusually resplendent creatures with bright blue and orange fins and bodies. And they fight—to the death—when challenged by anything their size. Don't worry, you are safe enough, even if you fall into some cere-monial pond where they are kept. You are more likely to incur the wrath of their owners than of the fish themselves.

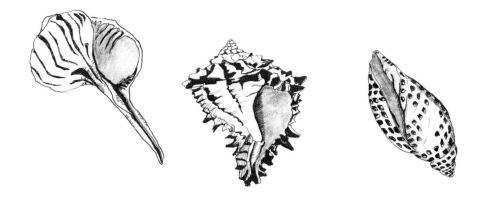

SHELLS

Shells, those sometimes massive, sometimes delicate external skeletons of various sea creatures, have been treasured for their beauty, used for coins and commerce, collected by idle sea coast strollers, and even used by industry in building materials.

Sea shells is a general name for three basic kinds of sea creatures: *Gastropods*, which are snails and snail-like animals that live in beautiful cone-shaped shells; *Pelecypoda*, which we know as clams, oysters, and scallops; and *Cephalopoda*, which includes the squid and the octopus. There are 50,000 varieties of these three general categories of sea animals, and each one has its own eccentricities. Some are deadly, some are shy, some have one foot, some have eight, some even change their sex halfway through their life!

There is no coast that does not have some evidence of sea shells, be they clinging barnacles on a rocky, beachless shore, or the resplendent oversized conches that bask like royalty on the sands of the South Pacific. Shells are beautiful, durable, plentiful, and available. They just lie on the sand waiting to be picked up! If beachcombing is your pleasure, follow these tips, and you will be able to collect some real deep-sea treasure of your own.

When engaging in serious shell collecting, bring along a net or mesh bag to hold your treasures. Two hands is never enough. Low tide is the best time to beachcomb. If you are at the shore during a full moon, the picking is particularly good. Since the tide comes in higher and ebbs out further then than at other times of the month, more shells than usual are brought onto the beach and more of the beach is exposed.

Immediately after a storm the shore is often littered with fragile and still living sea creatures. These shells will be brilliant in color because they have not been bleached by the sun or dried by the air. This is a good time to look for the unusual.

Snorkeling is a good way to locate less common species that live in shallow coastal waters.

If you want to preserve the shells you have collected, first soak the shells—particularly those that are closed—for 8 to 12 hours in a bleach solution. This will disinfect and remove any residue of animal matter or smell. Use baby or olive oil on the shells to keep them shiny and colorful.

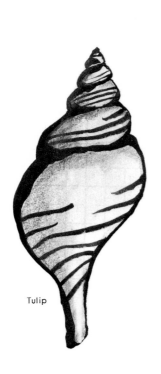

Tulip

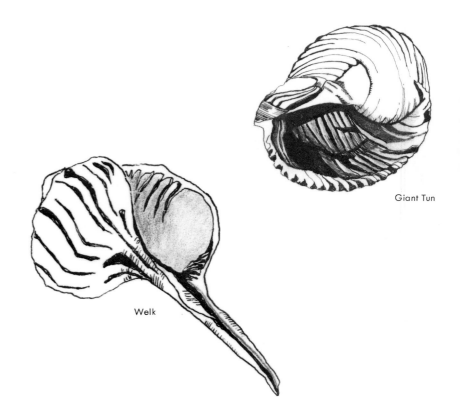

Giant Tun

Welk

TULIPS are a rare breed of meat-eating sea-shell animal. They feast on other mollusks. When looking for these, keep your eye out for bright orange, speckled with white. They are found throughout the South Atlantic.

WELKS are a large sea animal, sometimes up to 16 inches in length. Indians used their meat as food, their shells to make housewares, and sometimes even as weapons (either as projectiles or as sharp-edged club heads). You can find them in shallow waters and mud flats along the Gulf Coast and in Florida.

Despite their large size, a 7-inch GIANT TUN can be found washed up on the beaches in the Caribbean and southeast Florida. Live specimens live on underwater reefs. You will be able to recognize them by their distinctive ridged, curved top and the pale white inside color. (Other varieties are native to Panama and Peru.)

The SEA FAN, an underwater plant that often becomes hard when it dries out,

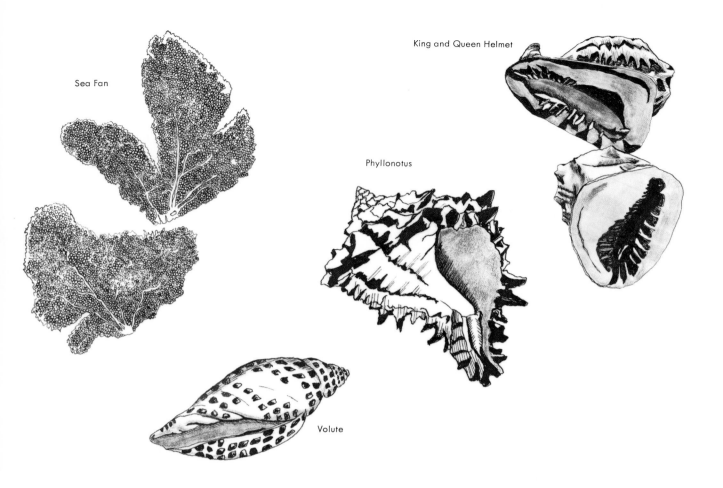

Sea Fan

King and Queen Helmet

Phyllonotus

Volute

is shell-like because it becomes mineral-filled—almost petrified, you might say. Don't step on it, it could cut your foot.

VOLUTES are hard to find and highly prized by collectors. A Peacock-tailed Volute, such as the one pictured here, once sold for $200. You'll have a chance to find this beach treasure if you are in southeast Florida—particularly Sanibel or Captiva Islands—and along the Georgia coast.

PHYLLONOTUS are a 3-inch-long meat-eating sea creature found in the tropical waters of South America, the Pacific coast of the U.S., and throughout the Pacific. It is distinctive because of its pointed dark-tipped spines.

The KING AND QUEEN HELMET shells look almost sharklike, with their gaping mouths and spiky white design. This particular variety grows up to 9 inches long and (with luck) can be found along the inlet shores of Japan, the Philippines, and the South Pacific, in southeast Florida, and the Caribbean, where the shell is often partially buried.

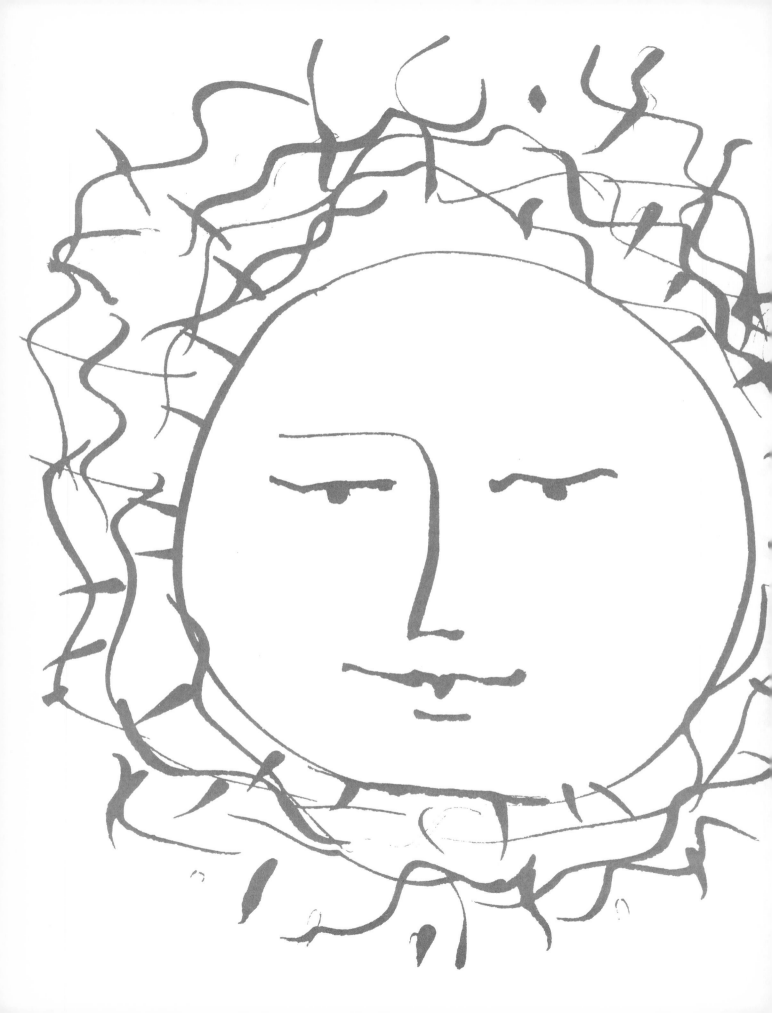

PART III
SUN SPOTS

12. Following the Sun

For most of human history, the idea of traveling a long distance (or even a short one) just to be in a sunny place would have been laughable—except for the fact that it would also have been unthinkable. True, the ancient Egyptians, the Incas of Peru, the Greeks of Rhodes, and many others worshipped the sun, but that was a matter of magical religion involving kings and deities, the regeneration of light and the fruitfulness of the earth.

But between ancient devotion to the sun as creator of life or father of kings and the modern phenomenon of burning Scandinavian flesh littering the beaches of southern Europe, there passed a long period when the sun was merely a facet of the environment, in moderation good for the crops but strictly to be avoided by the gentlefolk. For a tanned skin was the mark of a laborer, of one who toiled for his livelihood and earned his bread by the sweat of his brow. The upper classes wore masks and veils, were carried about in covered chairs and, later, in carriages. They cultivated fine white skins and languid ways. In eighteenth-century England ladies of fashion consumed small amounts of arsenic in order to give their complexions the highly prized blue-white finish. They apparently were unaware of arsenic's cumulative effect and ended as mortal sacrifices upon the altar of beauty.

It was the nineteenth century's romantic (as opposed to religious) worship of nature that brought about the total reversal of attitude that prevails today. Following the lead of the Romantic poets, the beautiful people of the day took to mooning over mountains, swooning over seas, and rhapsodizing over fields and forests. Spas and "cures" became popular. The health-restoring properties of mineral springs, ocean breezes, and pine-scented forests were highly regarded and, if these first tentative steps toward exposing oneself to the outdoors required that they take place in proximity to the reassuring shelter of a palatial hotel, so much the better. One could enjoy the outdoors but there was no question of one's being *forced* to be there because of economic necessity. On the contrary, it became a mark of wealth and style to live luxuriously and do nothing amid beautiful natural surroundings.

At the same time, attitudes toward the human body were beginning to change. Victorian prudery—which found a word like "legs" too coarse and substituted "limbs" even for pianos—was beginning to be supplanted by the growing influence of the health and fitness cults that emphasized physical exercise and exposure of the body to the strengthening effects of the elements. Sports became fashionable first as suitable pastimes for the leisure classes who had the time and money to indulge in them, and then as signs of success and status in the upwardly mobile middle classes. Women started to become involved in sports in the days when tennis was first exported to the world from Bermuda and was known as "spatchcock." Whether it was pleasure in physical activity or a good excuse to shed layers of constricting clothing that attracted women to sports is a moot point, but there is no question that from that time on it became fashionable at least to *look* as though one spent a great deal of time indulging in outdoor activities.

Since most of modern industrial society does not live in places where the sun shines all year long, living the outdoor life and maintaining the year 'round suntan are inextricably linked with travel. The whole concept of pleasure travel has, in fact, been changed by the desire for seasons in the sun. The traditional Grand Tour of art galleries and historical monuments could, after all, be followed at any time of year in appropriate places, but enjoyment of resort life and outdoor activities requires the right geographical location at the time of year.

Usually the most desirable situation involves a climate opposite to that found at home, both for relaxation and for snob appeal. For instance, the weather in the Caribbean islands is essentially the same all year 'round, but prices drop by half or more in the summer because it's the unfashionable season. Hordes of northern Europeans descend on Mediterranean coasts in winter, though many of them are only semi-sunny, because it's different from home and because that all-important tan (despite hazards discussed elsewhere in this book) must be nurtured to impress the stay-at-homes. Skiing in Switzerland in winter is fine, but skiing in South America in summer is overwhelmingly chic.

Thus, in this section, we have scoured a good part of the world to find more than two hundred great places to go that are beautiful, comfortable, and probably far away from where most of us live. We looked for the sun—sometimes tropical, sometimes not. We looked for wonderful places to stay—usually resort hotels, but sometimes city ones with unusual features; luxurious inns and lodges; even boats and barges and a super safari camp. We observed two major criteria in making our selections: luxury and variety. While no accommodations listed are lower than first class and most are deluxe, we realize that true luxury means different things to different people.

For some it means lavish hotels with many activities, much entertainment and socializing, casinos, nightclubs and dressing up as much as possible. Palm Beach, Monaco, the Costa del Sol, the Broadmoor in Colorado, the Cloister on Sea Island, Georgia, would all be good choices. Others want more unobtrusive luxury. They want beautiful surroundings, but little or no dressing up;

good food and service, but no ostentation. For them Little Dix Bay, Caneel Bay, Young Island, and Petit St. Vincent—all in the Caribbean—would fill the bill nicely as would Jenny Lake Lodge in Wyoming or the Kapalua Bay Hotel in Hawaii.

Then there are those who are beachcombers at heart. While not wanting to go utterly native, and certainly fond of basic creature comforts, still they want to feel unencumbered, unregimented and deliciously irresponsible. For them, Bonaire in the Netherlands Antilles, any Greek island, or yachting in the Grenadines present happily barefoot possibilities.

It has been said that Europeans, when they travel, expect to live worse than they do at home; Americans expect to live much, much better. In many ways, American standards seem to have prevailed and one can now expect private bathrooms in all hotels above a certain level—indeed, some of our selections provide "his" and "hers" or at least an extra lavatory. The swim-up bar in the middle of a swimming pool is an American innovation that has spread with lightning rapidity to all resort hotels that claim to be in the avant-garde (in Israel, with a largely non-drinking population, they have swim-up *snack* bars). Volleyball and bowling appear to be "in" sports in the Middle East and the Orient and trap and skeet shooting are remarkably ubiquitous.

Hotel practices concerning rates and meal service that developed as a result of local needs in different parts of the world have now been adopted internationally and standard terminology is used to identify them. World-wide, the most common system is European Plan (EP), which means that the hotel rate is for room only, with no meals. American Plan (AP) means that three meals a day are included in the room rate. This is the same as the European *pension* plan. Modified American Plan (MAP), similar to the European *demi-pension*, includes two meals (usually breakfast and dinner). There's a new wrinkle in some places, called Continental Plan (CP), which includes a light breakfast —usually pastry and beverage. Modified American Plan is probably the most popular in resort hotels nowadays since people tend to eat less than they used to and like to be free of meal schedules during the day. Full American Plan is becoming rare and is noted wherever it's available. Unless otherwise noted, it's generally safe to assume that a hotel operates on European Plan.

The descriptions that follow contain most of the facts that a traveler needs to know about hotels and destinations in some of the most attractive, exciting, sun-filled areas of the world. But we hope that readers will find more than facts, for we have tried to convey succinctly and impressionistically the specialness of each place—not only its specific features and activities, but also its flavor and ambience in a way that will bring together reader and resort in a happy leisure experience.

13. North America

THE NORTHEAST

Vermont has been synonymous with skiing since the days when the hardy skier expected nothing more luxurious than a rope tow and a bunk in a communal dormitory. Now the less-than-hardy can enjoy Poma lifts, double chair lifts, and elegant accommodations with French cuisine. But you can still find old-fashioned maple syrup, shining toylike villages clustered about a white-steepled church, and the indomitable Yankee character, as crisp and invigorating as an October morning in Vermont.

The Sugarbush Inn, Warren, Vermont 05674. Telephone: (802) 583-2301. A colonial-style country inn at the base of the Sugarbush ski area, offering comfortable accommodations ranging from spacious rooms to deluxe apartments and chalets. Sixteen tennis courts, modern teaching equipment, video playbacks. Challenge one of their 24 pros for a few sets. John Gardiner Tennis Clinics held weekly from June through September for total tennis experience. Robert Trent Jones-designed championship golf course. Airport with gliding and soaring; horses and polo; outdoor swimming pool; ski lifts; Cross Country Ski Center with miles of woodland trails starting at the inn's front door. International cuisine featuring Maine lobster and other New England specialties.

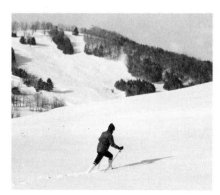

Woodstock, Vermont.

The Woodstock Inn, 14 The Green, Woodstock, Vermont 05091. Telephone: (802) 457-1100. Although the present building was constructed in 1969, an inn has stood on this spot in one of America's most picturesque villages since 1793. Traditional charm abounds in authentic touches—handmade patchwork quilts on the beds, antiques and local handicrafts, brass hinges, weathered Vermont timbers, hand-cut stone. In winter, logs blaze in a 10-foot fireplace. The inn operates two ski areas with trails for all talents, chair lifts, snowmaking equipment, Graduated Length Method of instruction. Ski Touring Center with over 40 miles of marked trails. Guests may use Woodstock Country Club facilities, including Robert Trent Jones-designed golf course with sand traps made of pure white Vermont marble powder, six clay and four all-weather tennis courts, and paddle tennis. Horseback riding nearby. Horse-drawn sleigh rides in winter, antiquing in nearby Vermont and New Hampshire countryside, exploring country stores and covered bridges, village strolling and hiking on marked trails. Fine cuisine typical of Rockresorts management.

THE SOUTH

To many Americans, their own southern states seem almost as foreign as odd corners of Europe, more foreign, perhaps, than many of the Caribbean islands that have become habitual vacation haunts for escapees from dreary northern winters. Landscape, food, architecture, language, customs and manners alert the senses to the awayness, the otherness of a land that is strange but evocative of numberless novels, plays, and films.

Within the sun-drenched South there is enormous variety to stimulate and satisfy a wide range of tastes, from the lushly antebellum *mise-en-scène* of pillared mansions framed in Spanish moss and semitropical gardens along the gulf coast of Alabama, to the far-reaching range of the Allegheny Mountains in West Virginia, which truly lives up to its name by combining the spirit of western expansion with the traditions of the Old South. But wherever you choose to relax in the American *mezzogiorno*, the one thread that runs consistently through the varied pattern is a courteous formality, stately as a minuet and just as gently anachronistic in the modern world. One luxurious seaside resort indulgently concedes that "hats and gloves are seldom seen" on its premises. The South is the place for ladies to look like ladies and gents to look like gents.

Grand Hotel, Point Clear, Alabama 36564. Telephone: (205) 928-9201. Five hundred wooded acres almost encircled by powdery white beaches lapped by the electric blue waters of Mobile Bay is the setting for the third Grand Hotel on this site since 1840. Golf is number one here—27 holes of championship calibre—but there is also swimming in the ocean and the 140-foot-diameter freshwater pool; a yacht basin with mooring for guests' boats; deep-sea and freshwater fishing; waterskiing, sailing in Rhodes Class 19 sailboats; ten tennis courts (regulation whites required); horseback riding; skeet and trap shooting; lawn bowling, volley ball; badminton; Ping-Pong and, if all else palls, croquet. Weather is glorious all year, and it can reach the high 70's in January, while breezes from Mobile Bay cool off the summers. Food specialties include Alabama Bon Secour oysters, blue crabs, and seafood gumbo. Shorts may be worn by men and women, but walking length only. Dinner is dressy but not formal, with dancing. In summer, beach luaus and steak fries with dancing under the stars.

The Cloister, Sea Island, Georgia 31561. Telephone (outside Georgia):

(800) 841-3223. Semitropical Sea Island is 10,000 acres of unspoiled land and marsh just off the coast of Georgia, halfway between Savannah and Jacksonville, Florida. The Cloister Hotel overlooks five miles of broad, firm beach. Eighteen tennis courts with all-weather Teniko surfaces (regulation whites required); 36 holes of golf on an oceanfront course; heated swimming pool; riding stables; skeet and trap shooting; hunting; fishing; boating; bicycling; lawn sports, and, of course, croquet. The mix of guests includes honeymooners, sportsmen, executives, and retirees. One of the few resorts still operating on full American plan, with seafood a specialty. Black tie on Thursdays, Saturdays, and nights of alfresco dinners.

Sea Pines Plantation, Hilton Head Island, South Carolina 29948. Telephone: (800) 845-6131. A private, 5000-acre community on Hilton Head Island, 45 miles northeast of Savannah, Georgia, part of the chain of offshore islands stretching along the eastern coast of the United States. Guests stay in fully furnished, privately owned homes or villa condominiums (with full hotel service) overlooking golf fairways, marshes, dense forests, or the Atlantic Ocean, or at the oceanfront Hilton Head Inn. Besides five miles of wide white beach, there are 72 holes of golf; more than 45 tennis courts; horseback riding; bicycle trails; yacht basin and marina; sailing; deep-sea and freshwater fishing; 14 swimming pools; and a 500-acre forest preserve. A wide variety of restaurants, many specializing in native seafood; nightspots with live entertainment and dancing; shops, boutiques, and art galleries. Great care has been taken to preserve the natural low-country beauty of the island.

The Greenbrier, White Sulphur Springs, West Virginia 24986. Telephone: (304) 536-1110. "Life as it should be" is the Greenbrier's motto, and there must be something to it, because vacationers have been coming to the area for nearly two centuries—originally to "take the waters" at the mineral-laden hot springs, but more recently to savor the crisp Allegheny mountain air, enjoy outdoor and indoor sports, and revel in nineteenth-century luxury combined with twentieth-century comfort. Facilities include 15 outdoor and 5 indoor tennis courts; platform tennis; three 18-hole

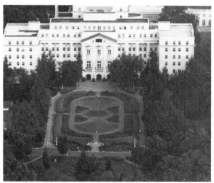

The Greenbrier, White Sulphur Springs, West Virginia.

golf courses; outdoor and indoor swimming pools; trap and skeet shooting; bowling; horseback riding on 200 miles of trails; carriage rides; archery; hiking; mineral baths, sauna and massage. The resort is known for friendly courtesy and lack of stuffiness as well as superb cuisine produced by graduates of its own culinary school.

Delta Queen and Mississippi Queen, The Delta Queen Steamboat Company, 511 Main Street, Cincinnati, Ohio 45202. When Mark Twain wrote about steamboating on the Mississippi, he said, "We were in the absolute South now. . . . The magnolia trees were lovely and fragrant . . . here the sugar region begins . . . and the plantations . . . were in view. . . . There was a tropical sun overhead . . . and a wide river hence to New Orleans." Aboard the beloved old Delta Queen, refurbished but elegantly Victorian, or the luxurious new Mississippi Queen—outwardly traditional, but with such interior amenities as all-weather climate control; a swimming pool, gym, and sauna; elevators; and a movie theater—history unfolds along the banks of the Mississippi from New Orleans to Natchez, Vicksburg, and, if you like, nearly to the river's source in northern Minnesota. Fine food and entertainment (with the emphasis on jazz, so close to its birthplace) and frequent side trips to beautifully preserved antebellum plantations, gardens, and landmark towns and villages are features of these cruises into the heart of the Louisiana Purchase.

FLORIDA

Florida stands alone as a resort destination, perhaps the best-known one in the world. *In* the South but not entirely *of* the South, the long sandbar peninsula washed by the Gulf of Mexico on the west, the Atlantic Ocean on the east, and the Caribbean Sea at its tip is the legendary site of the Fountain of Youth for which Ponce de Leon and other explorers searched in vain in the sixteenth century. Had they only known that in the twentieth century it would not be fountains, but Florida's endless beaches and languorous climate, enhanced by luxurious resorts and a profusion of outdoor sports, that would extend youth well beyond what any reasonable sixteenth-century man could have expected!

The Breakers, Palm Beach, 33480. Telephone: (305) 655-6611. The exterior design was inspired by the Villa Medici in Rome. The fountain in front was patterned after one in the Boboli Gardens in Florence. The lobby is reminiscent of the Palazzo Carega in Genoa. In all the public rooms, guests are surrounded by the Italian Renaissance. Thus is The Breakers aptly referred to as "the palace by the sea in Palm Beach." From the days when Consuelo Vanderbilt, Duchess of Marlborough, was a guest, to the present, when its Mediterranean Ballroom is the annual venue for Palm Beach's most fashionable ball, The Breakers has been redolent of fame, prestige, and, most definitely, fortune. Located on the oceanfront in the heart of Palm Beach, The Breakers provides two 18-hole golf courses, each with a clubhouse, pro shop, and driving range; 12 tennis courts; surf swimming from the private beach; outdoor saltwater pool and indoor freshwater pool; lawn sports; and

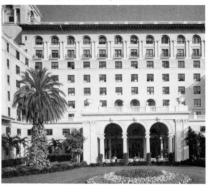

The Breakers, Palm Beach, Florida.

the scenic Lake Worth bicycle trail. Fine cuisine in palatial dining rooms and outdoor patios. Very convenient to Worth Avenue's fine shops.

Innisbrook Resort, Tarpon Springs, 33589. Telephone: (813) 937-3124. Primarily a golf and tennis resort, Innisbrook occupies a 1,000-acre heavily wooded wildlife sanctuary just south of the Greek-settled sponge diving and fishing community of Tarpon Springs and a short drive from Tampa International Airport. Accommodations consist of complete suites with kitchens and separate areas for entertainment. Innisbrook is a member of the Chaine des Rotisseurs, the international gourmet society. Dining facilities range from an elegant restaurant to a poolside snack bar. Activities include 63 holes of golf on three championship courses among 60 acres of natural lakes; 17 tennis courts and a major tennis program offering private lessons, clinics, and tournaments; swimming in five heated freshwater pools; lake fishing and sport fishing in the Gulf of Mexico; basketball and volleyball, sauna and exercise rooms; bicycling and sailing. Supervised programs for children.

The Key Biscayne Hotel and Villas, 701 Ocean Drive, Key Biscayne, Miami, 33149. Telephone: (305) 361-5431. On a private island minutes away from Miami International Airport, this oceanfront resort estate offers 101 hotel rooms plus 75 one-to-three-bedroom villas. On the property there are ten tennis courts (eight all-weather); an Olympic-size swimming pool; and an 18-hole Pitch-n-Putt golf course. Minutes away a 7,020-yard championship golf course (complimentary transportation provided). Distinguished cuisine in the Cape Florida Room, informal meals at the pool patio. Many guests stay a month or more.

South Seas Plantation, Captiva Island, 33924. Telephone: (813) 472-1551. A luxurious, low-key resort thirty miles from Fort Myers Airport. Bahamian-style villas and cottages for rent overlooking the beach and yacht basin as well as hotel suites with waterfront views and private sun decks in the antebellum Plantation House. Surf-free swimming beach; 12 tennis courts; 9 swimming pools; 9 holes of golf; offshore and charter fishing; and miles of excellent shelling beaches. Steve Colgate Offshore Sailing School operates from the deep-water

marina with courses for every level of sailing knowledge (and lack of knowledge). Three restaurants, jackets required in two of them after 6 P.M.

THE WEST

The West once meant cowboys and Indians, the howl of coyotes in the empty night, roughing it on the trail, panning for gold, ticky-tacky frontier towns springing up overnight and just as quickly falling into ruin when the gold or the silver ran out or the railroad right-of-way veered off in another direction. All this is the stuff of American folklore and mythology, that part of the national psyche that still searches for the wide open spaces of the next frontier.

The scenery is still grander and more colorful than life, the air of the mountains and the deserts still breathtakingly dry and clear, but out west has emerged a kind of luxury hardly to be matched in any other part of the country. No more ticky-tacky; western accommodations at the standard level are comfortable and attractive, at the luxury level, simply superb. Informality is admired, in manners as in clothes. Throw-it-away elegance is the hallmark of western chic—dinner jackets are a rarity, but finely crafted riding boots are worn with blue jeans and haute couture means high fashion sportswear.

The Arizona Biltmore, P.O. Box 2290, Phoenix, Arizona 85002. Telephone: (800) 261-8383. A fifty-year-old architectural landmark, much of the design inspired or actually done by Frank Lloyd Wright, this is the city's premiere resort for elegance and gracious service. Nestled into 1164 acres of date palms, citrus trees, flower gardens, and fountains, the sprawling 318-room, 4-story hotel is only a few miles from downtown Phoenix. In addition to the main building, there are individual cottages connected by landscaped walkways. Facilities include an Olympic-size swimming pool and health center; 27-hole championship golf course; 19 tennis courts (15 lighted for night play); riding stables and miles of private trails. Fine cuisine. European plan, modified American plan, and American plan available.

John Gardiner's Tennis Ranch, 5700 East McDonald Drive, Scottsdale, Arizona 85253. Telephone: (602) 948-

2100. Be forewarned: although this is a luxury resort, it is also "the West Point of tennis." There are swimming pools, golf, and horseback riding, but the *raison d'être* here is full-time tennis, with 24 courts and the most up-to-date training equipment. Seasoned travelers like the tennis clinics that are held from June to October.

The Wigwam, Litchfield Park, Arizona 85340. Telephone: (602) 935-3811. Low-lying buildings in the adobe hacienda style of the old Southwest, most accommodations at garden level with private entrances and patios. A completely self-contained resort with three championship golf courses; eight championship tennis courts and four practice courts equipped with teaching aids; oversized free-form swimming pool; horseback riding and desert breakfast rides; trap and skeet shooting; dancing and entertainment in the evening. Full American plan with varied cuisine, poolside buffet luncheons, twilight steak broils. The charming village of Litchfield Park is an extension of The Wigwam grounds, pleasant for strolling and shopping.

The Golden Door, P.O. Box 1567, Escondido, California 92025. Telephone: (714) 744-5777. To call this the aristocrat of American health spas is to understate the facts. It is the ultimate, the zenith, a true original, the most exquisite and expensive milieu for starvation in the world. But beautifully prepared, elegantly served, nutritionally sound starvation. Thirty pampered guests at a time are waited on, massaged, exercised, cosseted, and beautified by 87 devoted practitioners of the art of turning plump, tense, flabby bodies into slim, relaxed, lissome ones. It all takes place amid exquisite Japanese-derived decor and beautiful natural surroundings. Eight weeks of the year are for men only, four weeks for couples, and the rest of the year for women. Don't worry about what to wear; bring a bathing suit, heavy walking shoes, and caftan-type things for evening. The Golden Door will provide the rest.

La Costa Hotel & Spa, Rancho La Costa, Carlsbad, California 92008. Telephone: (714) 438-9111. The name tells it all: a self-contained resort 30 minutes by car from San Diego with a championship golf course (the annual PGA Tournament of Champions is played there); 25 tennis courts plus television-monitored

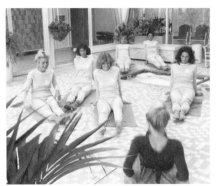
La Costa Hotel & Spa, Carlsbad, California.

practice alleys and teaching courts; Saddle Club with 21 miles of trails through spectacular country; four freshwater swimming pools; ocean swimming and deep-sea fishing five minutes away; and also separate spas for men and women that offer complete programs for weight reduction and physical fitness under medical supervision. Among the five restaurants on the premises, the Spa Dining Room is the one for calorie-controlled meals with no temptations.

La Quinta Hotel, La Quinta, California 92253. Telephone: (714) 564-4111. A Spanish-style luxury hotel in the desert at the foot of the Santa Rosa Mountains, 19 miles from Palm Springs, La Quinta is a 800-acre oasis of lawns, gardens, and date groves. Guest accommodations are in bungalows spaced far apart for privacy. Swimming pool, six tennis courts, horseback riding, 18-hole golf course at La Quinta Country Club. American plan, known for good food. Meals served in dining room, garden patio, or guest rooms.

Rancho Las Palmas Resort, Rancho Mirage, California 92270. Telephone: (714) 568-2727. Twelve miles south of Palm Springs, this new resort in early California style is in the midst of Rancho Las Palmas Country Club, giving guests access to 27 holes of golf and full golf clubhouse facilities as well as to 25 tennis courts and a tennis clubhouse. The two swimming pools have adjacent hydrotherapy pools. Guest rooms and villas overlook the golf course and man-made lakes.

The Tennis Club Hotel, 701 West Baristo Road, Palm Springs, California 92262. Telephone: (714) 325-1441.

One of the most expensively-built hotels in the world, with elegant, low-key ambience. Habitués very upper-crust, but not ostentatious. Tennis is the *only* game here (11 championship courts) and whites are the only garb on the courts. Billie Jean King was thrown out for wearing blue shorts. Swimming pool, three therapeutic hot pools, golf privileges at the Palm Springs Country Club.

Spa Hotel and Mineral Springs, 100 North Indian Avenue, Palm Springs, California 92262. Telephone: (714) 325-1461. Palm Springs really is built over mineral springs, which were used by the original Indian inhabitants, and most of the hotels have some form of therapeutic pool, but they use chlorinated water. The Spa Hotel, however, is built right over the original sacred Indian spring and uses the mineral water as it bubbles from the earth in its elaborate bath houses—pink and feminine for women, severely Spartan for men—both with individual terrazzo tubs, steam rooms, eucalyptus rooms, masseurs and masseuses. Incidentally, desert waters give off no unpleasant odor, it's lost through evaporation. Use of spa facilities is included in hotel rates, personal service is extra.

La Siesta Villas, 247 West Stevens Road, Palm Springs, California 92262. Telephone: (714) 325-2269. One- and two-bedroom villas with private walled-in patios in a lush tropical setting surrounding a spacious swimming pool. If you're so famous you can't stand the limelight anymore or have some other reason for wanting to be inconspicuous, this is the place to come. Absolute privacy is the rule. Every unit has a private telephone. Jascha Heifetz comes here to practice, Raquel Welch to sunbathe. This is where Alan Jay Lerner wrote the music for *Gigi* and producer Al Ruddy planned *The Godfather.* Some guests arrive by Lear jet, some don't, but owner Frank Merlo treats them all like friends and goes to great lengths to keep them happy.

Canyon Hotel Racquet & Golf Resort, 2850 South Palm Canyon Drive, Palm Springs, California 92262. Telephone: (714) 323-5656. Palm Springs' only private hotel golf course plus ten all-weather tennis courts and paddle tennis. Rooms and suites have lanais and mountain views. Three oversize swim-

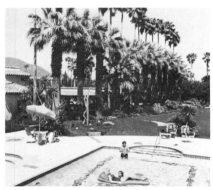

Canyon Hotel Racquet and Golf Resort, Palm Springs, California.

ming pools and Jacuzzis set in flowered courtyards, fully equipped spa, shaded bicycle paths. Fine dining in several restaurants, including poolside. Elegant shopping in hotel and nearby on South Palm Canyon Drive.

Note: The fashionable look in Palm Springs is casual and color-splashed. Pants, shirts, and sandals are the daytime rule for men and women. Sun cover-ups are a necessity. Women dress up at night, depending upon where they're going and what they think is appropriate for a desert desert. Russian sables have been seen, but a sweater is also protection against the cold night air. Men wear jackets and open-neck sport shirts. Only a very few private clubs require neckties, check when making reservations. And be sure to check on tennis attire—whites are required at The Tennis Club and at the private Racquet Club.

The Broadmoor, Colorado Springs, Colorado 80901. Telephone: (303) 634-7711. A palatial resort at the base of the Colorado Rockies since 1918, the Broadmoor has recently added Broadmoor West on the same property with balconied rooms and its own restaurant, swimming pool, and tennis courts. Few resorts can match the spectacular setting or the variety of activities available. Even though skiing begins in late November, golf is played the year around on three 18-hole championship courses; there are 16 all-weather tennis courts, two covered in winter by a heated, illuminated bubble; three heated swimming pools fed by mountain spring water; squash; boating; skeet and trap shooting; ice skating, hockey, and curling. Eleven eating and drinking rooms run the gamut from

Edwardian elegance to ski lodge informality around a copper-hooded fireplace. Wraps are necessary for summer evenings. Jacket and tie required in three of the dining rooms.

Tamarron, P.O. Box 3131, Durango, Colorado 81301. Telephone: (800) 525-5420. When *Avalanche,* starring Rock Hudson and Mia Farrow, was to be filmed, the script called for it to be set in "the most modern and luxurious Rocky Mountain resort." So it was filmed entirely at Tamarron, a stunning resort on 800 acres of rolling mountain terrain at an elevation of 7600 feet. Accommodations are in hotel suites or condominium apartments, most with working fireplaces and all with 20-mile views and luxurious appointments. Facilities include an 18-hole golf course carved into the mountainside; indoor and outdoor tennis; a 1000-foot ski run for hotel guests only; more challenging skiing at the Purgatory Ski Area, six miles away; indoor-outdoor swimming pool and health club; horseback riding; skeet and trap shooting; fishing; hunting; mountain climbing school; jeep and backpacking tours; wild river raft trips; ice skating; snowmobiling; sleigh rides; and supervised activities for children. Restaurants offer continental cuisine plus local game and mountain trout.

The Desert Inn, Las Vegas, Nevada 89109. Telephone: (800) 634-6906. It's been around for a while (Howard Hughes even holed up there for three years), but the newly reconstructed Desert Inn qualifies as this year's Las Vegas hotel and it's a dazzler—a deluxe self-contained resort in the middle of the Strip. Suites have *two* color television sets, onyx bathrooms, and ice makers or refrigerators. Other brand-new features are an Olympic-size swimming pool; large sundecks; ten outdoor heated Jacuzzis; a championship golf course and country club; five lighted tennis courts; a casino; nine restaurants; a showroom with top entertainment; and several cocktail lounges.

The other top Las Vegas hotels are Caesar's Palace, the Las Vegas Hilton and the MGM Grand—none of them shy about piling on the luxury. But unless you're a compulsive gambler who hasn't seen the sun in years, don't let the glamorous side of Las Vegas blind you to its other face—the spectacular desert

scenery that provides year-round recreation in the form of camping, boating, fishing, hiking, skiing, or just looking and admiring. Try a Scenic Airlines trip over Las Vegas and Hoover Dam, then *into* the Grand Canyon, flying its entire length below the rim. Or a spin over Vegas in a 1928 Ford Tri-motor—if you buy two tickets you can fly co-pilot!

The Bishop's Lodge, P.O. Box 2367, Santa Fe, New Mexico 87501. Telephone: (505) 983-6378. In the foothills of New Mexico's Sangre de Cristo Mountains, The Bishop's Lodge combines the luxury of a 1,000-acre resort with traditional New Mexican decor and the informality of the Old West just five minutes away from the heart of historic Santa Fe. Over 60 horses are available for trail riding in adjacent Santa Fe National Forest, with breakfast rides for the early birds and luncheon cookouts for late risers. There's a swimming pool and lawn sports, tennis complex, trap and skeet shooting, golf at Santa Fe and Los Alamos Country Clubs, and trout fishing in nearby mountain streams. Cuisine is American and international, with occasional Spanish specialties and steak fries. Dress is very informal, riding clothes are appropriate all day, jackets for evening.

Jenny Lake Lodge, P.O. Box 240, Moran, Wyoming 83013. Telephone: (307) 733-4647. A dozen craggy, cloud-high peaks thrust abruptly from the floor of Jackson Hole into the wide Wyoming sky. Here, in Grand Teton National Park, where Owen Wister wrote *The Virginian,* where *Shane,* a classic Western movie, was filmed, the vacationer may find secluded luxury in 30 individual log cabins at Jenny Lake Lodge. Reminiscent of the Old West, the cabins have all modern comforts and fine Rockresorts service. They border an alpine meadow just a few minutes' walk from lovely Jenny Lake, directly under the peaks of the towering Grand Tetons. In the valley are fine trout streams and miles of rustic trails for hikers and riders. Good food and service and the peace of a very private experience in nature set Jenny Lake Lodge apart from the usual frantic family chaos of the national parks. There is rafting down the Snake River, hiking, horseback riding, chuck wagon trips, golf, tennis, trout fishing, and swimming.

14. The Caribbean

North America's warm weather islands aren't all tucked neatly into the Caribbean Sea, as many people assume. Bermuda is in the mid-Atlantic on the same latitude as North Carolina. It's the Gulf Stream sloshing toward the British Isles that keeps it mild and green all year long. And the Bahamas start in the Atlantic near the coast of Florida, with the southernmost islands meandering into the Caribbean.

Nor do the islands resemble one another as much as many jaded travelers like to pretend they do. "If you've seen one island in the sun, you've seen them all," is a cocktail party chestnut that simply isn't true. Not true, at least, for the sensitive traveler who finds his pleasure in responding to the nuances of places and who delights in seeking out the differences in people and surroundings that make travel something more than just a change of climate.

The islands all have palm trees, beaches, and clear blue water. But some are windswept and bone-dry, like Bonaire and the Virgin Islands. Others, like Puerto Rico and Martinique, are jungle green with tropical rain forests. On islands that are, or were, British, dignity and good manners prevail, and English

is spoken in a variety of lilting accents, the most delightful perhaps being the Irish brogue of Barbados. French islands have good bread, a free hand with the wine, and bargains in perfume. And the people are as devoted to *la langue française* as any Parisian. Dutch islands are clean and tidy, with good beer and memories of another empire in the form of the frequently served rijsttafel. The Danes and the Swedes left only place names, but the Spanish influence still flourishes in Puerto Rico and Santo Domingo. Africa has touched most of the islands but left its stamp indelibly on Haiti.

BAHAMAS

Bargains in British goods and Bahamian handicrafts. Yachting center for motor more than sail, great sport fishing center. Active night life in Nassau and Paradise Island, strictly barefoot make-your-own fun in the Out Islands.

The Ocean Club, Paradise Island, P.O. Box N3707, Nassau. Cool, understated elegance. Plush accommodations, some villas with private pools. Secluded private beach, nine tennis courts, alfresco dining.

Ambassador Beach Hotel, Golf & Tennis Club, P.O. Box N3026, Nassau. Deluxe but not stuffy, active atmosphere, casino. Tennis, golf, swimming pool, restaurants plus access to all facilities at Balmoral Beach.

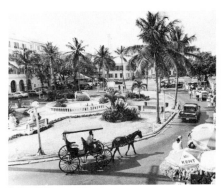

Rawson Square, Nassau.

Balmoral Beach Hotel, Golf & Tennis Club, P.O. Box N7528, Nassau. Stately British colonial, elegant and charming. Spacious accommodations, superb food. Beach and sports facilities plus access to additional ones at Ambassador Beach.

BERMUDA

As British as they come, and charming. Pink beaches, pastel cottages, white-helmeted policemen. Winters mild but not warm enough for swimming. Honeymooners galore, but popular with all ages, singles too. Plenty of nightlife if you look for it.

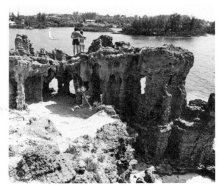

Ely's Harbor, Bermuda.

The Coral Beach and Tennis Club, South Road, Paget 6-01. On a cliffside with fabulous private beach, tennis, squash, 18-hole golf course. Introduction by member or former guest required.

Lantana Colony Club, Somerset Road, Sandys 9-02. Charming cottages in 20 acres of gardens. Private beach, pool, tennis, golf, sailing, fishing. Maid prepares breakfast in your own cottage, dining in garden solarium.

Mid Ocean Club, St. George's 1-22. Exclusive club on beautiful estate with large private beach. Tennis courts, championship golf course. Introduction by member required for accommodation and golf.

ANTIGUA (BRITISH WEST INDIES)

A friendly, green island with 365 unspoiled, uncrowded beaches and some of the best duty-free shopping in the Caribbean. Tennis Week is in January, Sailing Week in the spring, and Carnival Week erupts around the end of July. A haven for yachtsmen.

Curtain Bluff, P.O. Box 288. Fifty large double rooms with private outdoor terraces directly on bathing beach. Both

surf and calm sea bathing. Rates include sailing, waterskiing, skindiving and aqualung equipment, boating, tennis, and golf. Fine cuisine, extensive wine cellar.

Galley Bay Surf Club, P.O. Box 305, St. John's. Individual cottages really on the beach with private lanais and islandy decor. Slightly inland, Gauguin Village of native-style thatched huts in a coconut grove beside a salt lake. Casual, imaginative place. Rates include horseback riding, tennis, snorkeling, and fishing. Sailing, golf, and deep-sea fishing available.

Half Moon Bay Hotel, Box 144, St. John's. Ninety-eight oceanfront deluxe rooms with private patios or balconies on 150 acres facing Half Moon Bay. Enormous freshwater pool, championship tennis complex, scenic nine-hole golf course, sailing, snorkeling, scuba diving, deep-sea fishing. International cuisine, West Indian entertainment under the stars.

BARBADOS (WEST INDIES)

Never occupied by any power but Britain, and now independent, Barbados is proudly called "Little England" by its inhabitants, who maintain the stiff upper lip and innate good manners of the mother country. "The climate is what draws people here," says Oliver Messel, uncle of Lord Snowdon. "It's bracing, scintillating, refreshing and never humid." *That's* the kind of people who come to Barbados.

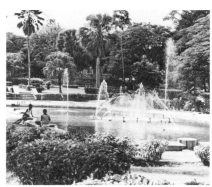

Barbados.

Sandy Lane Hotel, St. James. If you can't wangle an invitation as a guest in a private house, this is the next most fashionable place to stay. The hotel stands

amidst beautifully landscaped tropical gardens along, yes, a sandy beach. Continental cuisine plus Barbadian specialties, tennis, golf, water sports. Un-islandy decor, but plush and comfortable.

Coral Reef Club, St. James. Cottages and suites with private patios on the beachfront or in tropical gardens. Twelve beautiful acres with white sand beach. Fishing, sailing, skindiving. Can exchange dinners with other hotels. Pukka types often found here, retired major generals, a titled Englishman or two.

Cobblers Cove Hotel, St. Peter. Thirty-eight suites with living room, bedroom, kitchenette, and balcony or patio facing the beach or the gardens. Dining room is in a seaside castle left over from pirate days. Has played host to film and television luminaries and the prime minister of Quebec.

BONAIRE (NETHERLANDS ANTILLES)

A haven of tranquillity caressed by the trade winds but out of the hurricane zone, a sanctuary for flamingos and a paradise for divers, Bonaire is a superb place for doing absolutely nothing. There's room for only 300 tourists on this unspoiled island. Hotels are informal but comfortable.

Flamingo Beach Hotel. Individual cottages and seafront rooms with balconies (you can throw crumbs to the brilliantly colored fish), open-air dining room and local entertainment in this friendly little hotel, where coats and ties are strictly forbidden. Scuba diving and water sports.

Hotel Bonaire. Slightly larger, slightly livelier, with indoor dining, swimming pool, casino, large beach, tennis courts, scuba and water sports center.

BRITISH VIRGIN ISLANDS

Quiet and lovely, with varied terrain, the British Virgin Islands are far less developed for large- or even medium-scale tourism than their American cousins. Resorts are small and informal, blending easily into the environment without disturbing the natural beauty of their surroundings.

Little Dix Bay, Box 70, Virgin Gorda. One of the world's most beautiful resorts. Just 66 rooms in cone-topped cottages with private terraces curled around a great crescent beach in an idyllic South Seas setting. Excellent meals served outdoors in the dramatic central pavilion facing the beach. Tennis, horseback riding, sailing, waterskiing, fishing, snorkeling, and scuba diving. No telephones, plenty of hammocks. Rockresorts management.

Peter Island Yacht Club, P.O. Box 211, Roadtown, Tortola. An attractive Scandinavian hotel and village resort with two palm-fringed beaches. Beach bar, swimming pool, tennis, anchorage and marine facilities.

Marina Cay Hotel, P.O. Box 76, Roadtown, Tortola. A charming cottage hotel on a six-acre island with a well-protected anchorage and a first-rate snorkeling reef. Private beach, terrace dining, sailing, fishing, scuba diving.

DOMINICAN REPUBLIC

Occupying two-thirds of the island of Hispaniola, this is where Columbus bumped into the new world in 1492. Sometimes called the best-kept secret in the Caribbean, the Dominican Republic has a pleasant tropical climate, friendly people, good beaches, and interesting Spanish ambience. Amber, the national gem, is a good buy, as are cigars, mahogany objects, and paintings.

Casa de Campo, Villas & Country Club, La Romana. Rustic and tranquil, with a private jet-strip and a polo field. Also *casitas* with stunning decor by Dominican native Oscar de la Renta, moonlight sailing, golf, tennis, horseback riding, and swimming at a hidden beach. Jetsetters, like Lee Radziwill, Cheryl Tiegs, and Dino de Laurentiis zoom in to unwind at this contemporary Garden of Eden.

Hotel Santo Domingo, Santo Domingo. Set in 14 acres of gardens overlooking the Caribbean, this is the place to stay for sightseeing and shopping in the nation's capital city. Elegantly Dominican interior by Oscar de la Renta, swimming pool, tennis, sophisticated dining.

GRENADA (BRITISH WEST INDIES)

The original "spice island," it still exports aromatic nutmeg and cloves. Dra-

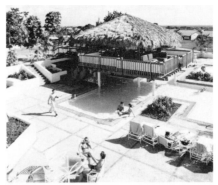

Casa de Campo, Dominican Republic.

matic mountainous scenery, exotic flowers. Black volcanic sand beaches on one side, white coral sand on the other side. Picturesque St. George's harbor a mecca for yachtsmen. Remember this is British, not Spanish, so call it Gre-NAY-da.

Secret Harbour Hotel, L'Anse aux Epines. Mediterranean-style cottages with living rooms and terraces facing the water, five miles from St. George's. Antique furnishings, Italian tile baths. Small sandy beach, swimming pool, tennis, water sports, sport fishing, yacht charters. West Indian buffet on Sundays, local lobster a specialty.

GUADELOUPE (FRENCH WEST INDIES)

Two islands—Basse-Terre and Grande-Terre—joined by a drawbridge form this butterfly-shaped *département* of France, where an appealing Creole culture has emerged out of French and African strains. Strictly French-speaking (except in the largest hotels), it's a tropical corner of the old country. Some of the best prices anywhere for French products, especially perfume. On August 12 everyone turns out for the Fête des Cuisinières to honor the island's women cooks and indulge in a free five-hour banquet (invitations available through hotels). Women dress up at night, men dress down. Charming nearby islands for side trips.

Auberge de la Vieille Tour, Gosier. Comfortable old-style hotel centered around an old sugar mill in acres of tropical gardens. Balconied rooms on terraced hillside leading to private beach. Tennis, water sports, deep-sea fishing,

freshwater pool. Excellent cuisine, international clientele.

The Hamak, St. François. Cottages and villas strung along the beach or overlooking the marina on a 250-acre estate. Tropical gardens, air strip, Robert Trent Jones golf course. Tennis, bocce ball, waterskiing, sailing, windsurfing, snorkeling and greens fees included in rates. Deep-sea fishing, flying lessons, and excursions available. Luxury in a casual, unspoiled setting, privacy, and haute cuisine with complimentary wine.

HAITI

One-third of the island of Hispaniola, the hemisphere's oldest black republic. Gentle, friendly people who treasure their French language as well as their unique Creole culture with its own tongue. Dramatic tropical scenery. Warm at sea level, as cool as San Francisco in the high country. Good beaches, but difficult to get to. Remarkable literary culture, influenced by France, and a musical one, almost purely African. Superb painting and sculpture, Port-au-Prince art galleries a must for the visitor.

Habitation Leclerc, Port-au-Prince. If you can wallow in supreme luxury without twinges of guilt, try this 30-acre oasis on the estate of Napoleon's notorious sister, Pauline Bonaparte Leclerc. Elegantly appointed villas perched on a hillside, round bathtubs you can swim in, tennis, horseback riding, and swimming pools. Good service and privacy in flawless surroundings. No children allowed.

El Rancho Hotel, Port-au-Prince. A sprawling estate in the Boutillier Mountains, 1200 feet above Port-au-Prince and its harbor. Large, beautifully decorated rooms with balconies or terraces, alfresco dining, strolling guitarists by the pool. Two swimming pools, a whirlpool, pool bar under a waterfall, championship tennis, badminton, gymnasium, saunas, and outdoor backgammon club.

Grand Hotel Oloffson, Port-au-Prince. An oddity in the hotel world. Literary and theatrical greats have long been attracted to this specimen of gingerbready Victoriana, almost obscured by tropical foliage at the very edge of town. John Gielgud, Lillian Hellman, Anne Bancroft, James Jones, Marlon Brando, and Irving Stone have had rooms named after them. It's cool and breezy, with great views, a swimming pool, convenient transportation. The owners don't answer mail and service tends to be erratic.

JAMAICA (WEST INDIES)

A large island, mountainous and green, cool at high altitudes, warm but breezy at sea level. The birthplace of reggae, with exciting music and swinging nightlife in Montego Bay and Kingston. Montego is the tourism capital, but elegant Ocho Rios is growing fast. Plenty to see and do—plantation tours, river rafting, cricket matches, innumerable beaches. Shop for art, handicrafts, and designer fashions, especially "Kareebas," a men's coat that evolved here.

Round Hill Hotel, Montego Bay. An international favorite, exclusive but informal and friendly. Rooms with private balconies and lush villas with private pools scattered on a peninsula sloping down to a perfect crescent beach. Water sports, spear fishing, tennis, boating, horseback riding. Golf nearby.

Royal Caribbean, P.O. Box 167, Montego Bay. A lovely old hotel, one of the first to be built in Montego Bay. Graciously elegant, every room just a few steps from the white sand beach or the huge free-form pool, all with private patio or living porch. Tennis, water sports, golf nearby. Dress usually informal, jackets only for Saturday and Sunday evening dining.

Jamaica Inn, Ocho Rios. Some call it swanky, some call it stodgy, but the buildings and grounds are among the loveliest in Jamaica. Located on a secluded beach. Freshwater pool and croquet court, golfing at nearby country club. British and Canadian industrialists favor it.

Jamaica Association of Villas and Apartments, Ocho Rios P.O. For a truly luxurious vacation, renting a Jamaican villa may be the answer. Villas range from simple to palatial and come with cooks, maids, and butlers. It's a wonderful way to do your own thing without having to do anything. J.A.V.A. has offices in New York, Chicago, Los Angeles, Miami, Quebec, Toronto, and London.

MARTINIQUE (FRENCH WEST INDIES)

An island of flowers and super sunshine spiced with Creole charm. French to the fingertips and a full-fledged *département* of *la patrie,* 4,000 miles away. Columbus called it "the best, richest, sweetest, most charming country in the world." France exchanged Canada for it along with Guadeloupe. And, of course, its most famous historical figure is the Empress Josephine, born on a sugar plantation and commemorated all over the island. Fantastic shopping for French goods— Roger Albert in Fort-de-France is the cheapest place in the world for perfume (pay with traveler's checks, credit cards —anything but cash—for the lowest prices).

Hotel Plantation de Leyritz, Basse-Pointe. An elegant hotel in the midst of a working banana plantation on a breezy mountainside near Mont Pelée. Modern conveniences along with the graciousness of a 200-year-old residence with marble and tile floors, antique furnishings, and romantically decorated rooms and bungalows. Traditional French and Creole cuisine. Swimming pool, tennis, horseback riding. Beach is 18 miles away, transportation furnished once a day. They claim that English is spoken, which makes one suspicious.

Hotel la Batelière, Fort-de-France. Closest resort hotel to Fort-de-France, on a promontory with a small beach. All rooms with balcony. Indoor and outdoor dining, casino, discotheque, and folklore shows. Swimming pool, tennis, water sports, deep-sea fishing, cruising on 58-foot ketch.

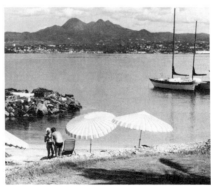
Martinique.

Hotel Bakoua Beach, Pointe du Bout. Traditional family-owned hotel on the beach. Rooms with balcony or patio at water's edge or on hillside. Beach snack bar, swimming pool, tennis, water sports, golf, and horseback riding nearby. Dinner dancing, Ballets Martiniquais on Fridays.

PUERTO RICO

It's always summer in Puerto Rico, a tropical island with a zip code. A United States commonwealth, it's superficially very American, especially in San Juan, but out on the island the Spanish influence prevails, and English is spoken only sporadically. It's a major air transport hub for most of the Caribbean.

Palmas del Mar, Humacao. A cluster of five pastel-colored villages only an hour's drive from San Juan, but light-years away in peaceful ambience. All vaguely Mediterranean—one like a fishing hamlet in the south of France for boating enthusiasts, another like an Italian hill town for tennis players, one for golfers, one right on the beach. Villas have living rooms and kitchens with all modern appliances, hotel rooms at the exquisite 23-room Palmas Inn are spacious and have private terraces overlooking the Caribbean. Sporting facilities available to all guests. Formal restaurant, poolside terrace dining, sidewalk cafe, and swim-up bar.

Dorado Beach Hotel, Dorado Beach. A 1000-acre tropical beach resort 20 miles west of San Juan, with two outstanding seaside golf courses, two miles of ocean beaches, and its own private airport. Swimming pools, tennis courts, hiking, bicycling, lawn games, dinner dancing, air tours to nearby islands. Extremely comfortable, imaginative construction and decor using indigenous style and color.

ST. MARTIN/ST. MAARTEN

A charmingly schizophrenic little island, half-French, half-Dutch, that lives in happy coexistence with itself. The Dutch part is more developed touristically and has the big international airport, the cruise ship pier, casinos, and much duty-free shopping. The French side has quaint little towns, open markets, seaside cafes, excellent restaurants, an unhurried pace, and the only nudist beach on the otherwise conservative island.

La Samanna, Boite Postale 59, 97150 St. Martin, French West Indies. Reputed to be the poshest place in the entire

Caribbean. A descending crescent of whitewashed villas on 4000 feet of magnificent beach. Moorish-Mediterranean decor, fine French and Creole cuisine, superb informality. Swimming pool, tennis, snorkeling, waterskiing, sailing.

Le Galion, Baie de l'Embouchure, St. Martin, French West Indies. Quiet and comfortable on two mile-long beaches. Nudist beach five minutes away. Excellent snorkeling along reef, tennis, fishing, waterskiing. Good French cuisine.

Oyster Pond Yacht Club Hotel, P.O. Box 239, Philipsburg, St. Maarten, Netherlands Antilles. Small and plush, built of stone and whitewashed stucco, it stands at the end of its own green peninsula above a half mile of pure white beach. Twenty individually decorated rooms, each with balcony and water view. Reef-protected water for swimming and snorkeling, tennis courts, marina and yacht club. International cuisine with Creole touches, outdoor dining.

The Caravanserai, P.O. Box 113, St. Maarten, Netherlands Antilles. Built in hacienda style on its own peninsula with excellent beach, fresh- and saltwater pools, tennis, golf nearby. Dining room open to the breezes, rijsttafel buffet on Wednesdays, barbecue with local specialties on Sundays. Butlers and chauffeurs available.

ST. VINCENT AND THE GRENADINES (BRITISH WEST INDIES)

The Grenadines are a chain of 32 sparkling islands and cays stretching from St. Vincent to Grenada, with their capital at Kingstown on St. Vincent. The finest yachting area in the eastern Caribbean— some say in the world. White sand beaches abound and small hotels—simple or sumptuous—are the rule. Carnival on St. Vincent, just before Lent, is the climax of the year—lavish but uncommercialized, spontaneous fun for everyone. Don't pass up a chance to go to a "jump-up" (dance)—magnificent dancing often based on old European forms, courtly manners, and a friendly mix of locals, hotel guests, and visiting yachtsmen.

Petit St. Vincent Resort, The Grenadines. Correspondence and inquiries to

Petit St. Vincent, P.O. Box 12506, Cincinnati, Ohio 45212. A privately owned out-island with superb white sand beaches and crystal-clear water in a lagoon surrounded by a horseshoe reef. Twenty-two separate cottages, each a suite with living room and patio, built of native volcanic rock and exotic South American woods. Run like a private club with well-trained staff. Fine cuisine, sailing, snorkeling, scuba, tennis—but mainly serene relaxation.

Young Island, St. Vincent. An island off an island, 200 yards offshore from St. Vincent, reached by water taxi. Fifteen individual thatched-roof cabanas with private patios. The island is a tropical garden with hammocks strung along the beach under their own thatched roofs, Carib canoes, sailfish and snorkeling gear to use. *Shoes are not worn* (unless you insist on them for tennis). Women dress for dinner, men don't. Delicious local cooking, a floating bar you have to swim to, daily sailing trips to nearby islands.

TRINIDAD AND TOBAGO (WEST INDIES)

Two islands that comprise the most cosmopolitan country in the West Indies, with a mix that includes Africans, East Indians, Europeans, French, Spanish, Portuguese, Lebanese, Syrians, Chinese, and North and South Americans. Trinidad, the birthplace of calypso, is spectacular at Carnival time, has great shopping in Port-of-Spain. Tobago, reputed to be Robinson Crusoe's island, floats idyllically in the sea, rimmed by peaceful golden beaches.

Trinidad Hilton, Port-of-Spain, Trinidad. The upside-down Hilton where you go *down* to your balconied room overlooking the sea, mountains, and Queen's Park Savannah. A Trinidad-shaped swimming pool, sunken bar with calypso entertainment, West Indian and international cuisine in the restaurant built around a buccaneer-style smoke oven. Golf, beaches, tennis and boating nearby.

Arnos Vale Hotel, P.O. Box 208, Scarborough, Tobago. Cottages and suites for 54 guests meander down to the beach on a lush 400-acre estate. Swimming pool, snorkeling in crystalline reef waters, and big game fishing. Excellent cuisine

with West Indian specialties and select wine list. Odd but charming touches are Murando chandelier and Pleyel grand piano built for the Paris Exhibition of 1851.

UNITED STATES VIRGIN ISLANDS

Three lovely islands, once Danish, now American: bustling St. Thomas for shopping and nightlife; sedate, green St. Croix, noted for golf; and dreamy little St. John, mainly left to nature as a national park.

Caneel Bay Plantation, P.O. Box 120, Cruz Bay, St. John, 0083. Blending easily into its environment on a peninsula rimmed by seven talcum-soft white beaches and transparent blue water, Caneel has a unique international cachet for informal luxury, Rockresorts cuisine, and superb water sports. Most accommodations right on the beach, but choose those on the low cliffs and headlands for constant breezes. Scuba, snorkeling, boating, deep-sea fishing, tennis, hiking in the national park. Pollen-free air. At night, casual dress-up for women; jackets, no ties, for men.

Sugarbird Beach and Tennis Club, Box 5157, Water Island, St. Thomas, 00801. A resort hideaway on an island seven minutes from Charlotte Amalie. Beautiful beach, swimming pools, all water sports, sailing, and tennis.

Gentle Winds Beach Resort, St. Croix, 00801. Spacious air-conditioned villas and suites with living rooms, kitchens, and terraces overlooking sea or mountains. Beachfront restaurant. Tennis courts, private beach, freshwater pool, championship golf course nearby, excursions to Buck Island underwater park.

St. Tropez Charters, Ltd., St. Thomas. Correspondence to 21 School Street, Boston, Massachusetts 02108. Sailing school vacations with highly qualified instructors or bareboat charters —everything provided including food and menus for doing it all on your own. Fleet consists of Pearson 365's and C&C Landfall 42's with auxiliary diesel engines. Great sailing waters among the legendary 11,000 Virgin Islands, hasn't been a hurricane in over 50 years, always land in sight.

15. Mexico, Central and South America

MEXICO

Mexico, the United States' nearest truly foreign destination, has something for everybody. Spectacular ruins, smooth white beaches, charming Spanish colonial towns, swinging night life, unique handicrafts, unusual cuisine, a cultural amalgam of the old world and the new—every visitor can find an aspect of the country that appeals to his own tastes.

Hotel Las Brisas, P.O. Box 281, Acapulco. Privacy attracts celebrities to the 250 *casitas,* each with a private or semiprivate pool sprinkled with fresh hibiscus blossoms, on a hillside overlooking Acapulco Bay. No lobby, pink jeeps deliver breakfast to the *casitas* and transport guests up and down the hill. If privacy palls, there's La Concha Beach Club with two saltwater pools, tennis, backgammon, waterskiing, sailing, and skin diving.

Rancho La Puerta, Tecate, Baja California. Mailing address: Tecate, California 92080, USA. A low-pressure spa resort founded by the owners of The Golden Door in California. Bracing climate and unspoiled natural surroundings,

35 miles from San Diego. Exercise or not, as you like. Spa and sports facilities include tennis, swimming pools, hot therapy pool, saunas, nine gyms, volleyball, backgammon, putting greens, hiking trails, Swedish massage, herbal wraps, facial treatments, 1000-calorie-a-day diet.

Hyatt Baja, Apartado 12, Cabo San Lucas, Baja California Sur. Stunning Indian pueblo-style buildings clustered around plazas on cliffs overlooking the Sea of Cortez in the fishing capital of the world. Private beach, three-tiered swimming pool with sunken bar, tennis, backgammon, deep-sea fishing, scuba diving, snorkeling, sailing, horseback riding, hunting.

Hotel Twin Dolphin, Cabo San Lucas, Baja California Sur. Set high on a bluff overlooking secluded beaches, ultramodern private *casitas* surrounded by desert landscaping. Freshwater swimming pool with swim-up bar and waterfalls encircled by dining terraces; tennis, snorkeling, scuba diving, sailing, and waterskiing, backgammon, 18-hole putting green, trap shooting, and, most important, deep-sea fishing.

Hotel El Tapatio, Boulevard Aeropuerto No. 4275, Guadalajara, Jalisco. Pueblo-style terrace suites in seven tiers encircle a hill overlooking Mexico's second city. "Pleasure plateau" at the top has swimming pool, restaurants, bars, sauna, children's playground, backgammon area. Eight clay tennis courts, putting green, horseback riding, bullring, four golf courses nearby.

Hotel Ixtapan, Nueva Ixtapan, State of Mexico. Mexico City office, Paseo de la Reforma 132, Mexico City 6, D.F., Mexico. A luxurious resort spa with hot mineral springs and private thermal baths 75 miles from Mexico City. Swimming pools, horseback riding, gymnasium, tennis, golf, health and beauty institute, men's health club. Rest and tranquillity or plenty of activity, as you like.

Las Hadas, Manzanillo, Colima. One of the world's most lavish resorts, an Arabian fantasy of whitewashed minarets, cupolas and mosquelike domes. Hanging gardens clamber over villas and ornamental towers. Sugary sand beach with Moorish beach tents, two swimming

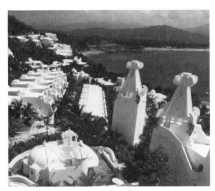

Las Hadas, Manzanillo, Mexico.

pools with islands and waterfalls, tennis, golf, private marina, deep-sea fishing. International cuisine in open-air, terrace, and indoor restaurants.

Hotel Camino Real, Mariano Escobedo 700, Mexico 5, D.F. The only complete resort hotel in the heart of Mexico City and a social center for the city. Swimming pools, tennis courts, seven-and-a-half acres of gardens, ten restaurants, bars and nightclubs, including Fourquet's de Paris for French cuisine.

Posada Vallarta, Puerto Vallarta, Jalisco. Liz and Dick transformed Puerto Vallarta from a sleepy fishing village into a mecca for tourists, but Posada Vallarta is unspoiled and picturesque, with colonial charm and sophisticated service. Private balconies, fine beach, deep-sea fishing, tennis, hunting, horseback riding, waterskiing, skin diving, polo on donkey back. Mexico and continental cuisine, indoor and outdoor dining.

Hotel-Club Akumal Caribe, Akumal, Yucatan. Facing the crystal-clear water of the Caribbean in a garden of hibiscus and wild orchids, Mayan villas and luxury bedrooms. Some of the world's best skin diving, snorkeling, scuba diving, and bird watching. Fresh seafood and Mayan specialties. Near the ruins of Cobá and the ancient Mayan city of Tulum.

CENTRAL AMERICA

Hotel Contadora, Contadora Island, Panama. A deluxe 210-room ocean-front resort on one of the 13 white sand beaches of a 220-acre island gem in the clear waters of the Pearl Island Archipelago, 15 air minutes south of Panama City. Swimming pools, night-lighted tennis, nine-hole golf, deep-sea fishing, water sports, marina, casino, and shopping center.

SOUTH AMERICA

South America has long been a sleeping giant in the world of tourism, a vast treasure-house of barely-tapped riches for the traveler. Few places have adequate accommodation and transportation is sometimes sketchy, but development is coming, and there are already harbingers of enormous possibilities for the future.

ARGENTINA

Hotel Llao Llao, Bariloche. Pronounced "Jao Jao," it's a luxury hotel with rustic charm in this famous summer skiing area, right in the center of town with a casino. The town, reminiscent of a small European ski resort, is 15 minutes from the slopes of Cerro Cathedral, 3000 feet above sea level with its peak at 6000 feet. Average snow ranges from two feet at the bottom to nine feet at the top. Cable car, chair lifts, T-bars and rope tows. Maximum ski run two-and-a-half miles, vertical drop 3000 feet.

BRAZIL

Hotel Das Cataratas, Iguassu Falls. A handsome, sprawling hotel in traditional style overlooking the 200-foot plunge of the Parana River in 32 separate falls. The roar can be heard 15 miles away. If that's not enough water, there's a free-form swimming pool. Wildly spectacular scenery.

Tropical Hotel Manaus, Manaus. South America's largest resort hotel complex 1000 miles up the Amazon River amid thousands of acres of lush forest. Gracious colonial architecture, low and colonnaded, with spacious guest rooms. Tennis, mini-golf, two swimming pools, sauna with physiotherapy and massage, fishing, waterskiing, rafting, canoeing.

Tropical Hotel Tambau, Joao Pessoa. Ultra-modern, like a flying saucer right on the beach at Joao Pessoa in northeast Brazil. All rooms have a view

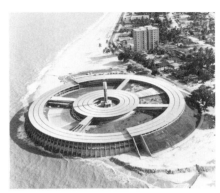

Tropical Hotel Tambau, Brazil.

of the sea or fabulous inner gardens. Swimming pools and shopping center.

Hotel Nacional, Gavea Beach, Rio de Janeiro. A city resort in a tall, cylindrical glass tower with panoramic views of the city, the sea and the mountains. Exceptional restaurants, nightclub with Carnival atmosphere. Swimming pools, sauna, golf, beach. Convenient for Rio sightseeing.

CHILE

Hotel Portillo, Portillo. Ski here in late July and August, when there's a hard base of 18 feet with 2 to 4 inches of powder cap. Hotel, 10,000 feet above sea level beside Lake Inca, is a self-contained resort with restaurants, nightclub, theater, and ski shops. Most slopes are expert and intermediate, three trails for beginners and two cross-country trails.

ECUADOR

Galapagos Islands. Information from Galapagos Tourist Corporation, 888 Seventh Avenue, New York, New York 10019. From Guayaquil comfortable cruise ships make four- to seven-night trips to the fascinating islands where Darwin made some of his most important discoveries. Only 80 people at a time may visit the islands in order to preserve their unspoiled quality. Animals are unique in the world and incredibly unafraid of people. All ships are air conditioned with all outside cabins and private bathrooms and carry trained nature guides.

16. Europe

AUSTRIA

In winter, most of Austria is one big ski resort. Small inns and guest houses are the rule, rather than large self-contained resort hotels. Hotels are clustered in the little towns surrounded by mountains and usually share facilities. Good food, gemütlichkeit and après-ski activity abound.

Hotel-Restaurant Goldener Adler, Innsbruck, Tirol. A historic Tyrolean inn founded in 1390, located in the Old Town pedestrian zone. Over the years kings and poets have stayed here, and it still offers first-class comfort and food.

Hotel Schloss Lebenberg, Kitzbuhel, Tirol. Beautiful international class hotel with complete spa facilities: underwater ray massage, mud baths, intensive sun treatment, ultraviolet rays, solarium, sauna, special diet by request. Tennis, curling, kindergarten.

Hotel Gasthof Post, Lech am Arlberg. A rustic Tyrolean-styled 300-year-old inn with antique furniture and modern comforts. Indoor swimming pool, sauna and massage, ice skating, curling, sleigh-riding, cross-country trails.

Hotel Schwarze Adler, St. Anton, Tirol. First-class hotel dating back to

1750, with a cozy atmosphere. Charmingly painted facade. Good restaurant and wine cellar. Swimming pool, curling, ice skating, sleigh riding.

Hotel Arlberg-Hospiz, St. Christoph am Arlberg, Tirol. A traditional inn 600 years old, with indoor swimming pool, sauna, nightclub, kindergarten. Curling, ice skating, sleigh riding.

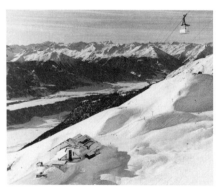

Innsbruck, Austria.

Alpenhof Sporthotel, Zurs, Arlberg. Elegantly simple Austrian-style with magnificent wood carving. Indoor swim-

ming pool, fitness room, massage and solaria, sun terrace. All ski trails end at the hotel entrance.

Hotel Alpenrose-Post, Zurs am Arlberg, Tirol. Good modern hotel with an international clientele. Indoor swimming pool, sauna and massage, outdoor snow bar, ski repair shop. Tea dancing.

FRANCE

France has everything, as we all know, but for sun-seekers there are three principal areas: the Côte d'Azur along the Riviera; the Basque coast, especially Biarritz; and the Alpine ski villages that range from simple to swinging. Whichever you choose, there will be superb food and wine and an unmistakably Gallic touch of elegance.

La Réserve de Beaulieu, 5 Boulevard General-Leclerc, 06310, Beaulieu-sur-Mer. The quiet atmosphere of a private residence with the luxury of a great hotel. Fifty guest rooms overlooking the sea, swimming pool, water sports, tennis and golf nearby, two-star winter and summer restaurants.

Hotel du Palais, 64200 Biarritz. Former residence of Napoleon III and Empress Eugénie, magnificently decorated and furnished. Swimming pool. Nearby: casinos, golf links, horseracing, bullfighting, tuna fishing, folklore shows and dances, musical events, formal social activities.

Hotel le Cagnard, rue Pontis Long, 06800 Cagnes-sur-Mer. An ancient Provençal house built on the ramparts of the medieval city of Haut-de-Cagnes between Nice and Cannes, two kilometers inland. Fishing, golf, and horseback riding nearby. Fine cuisine, interesting decor.

Hotel Carlton, La Croisette, Boite Postale 155 06403 Cannes. World-renowned *grande dame* of hotels in the center of the Croisette facing the Mediterranean. Elegant restaurant with terraces, good sand beach. Two minutes walk to Cannes Festival and Convention Complex.

La Residence du Cap, 161, Boulevard J-F Kennedy, 06600 Cap d'Antibes. Peaceful manor house in a large park on the peninsula of Cap d'Antibes. Swimming pool surrounded by palm trees, waterskiing, fishing, horseback riding, golf.

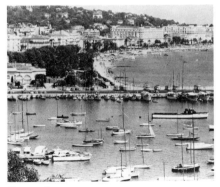

Cannes, France.

Hotel du Cap-Eden Roc, Boulevard J-F Kennedy 06604 Antibes. Fashionable, only 90 rooms, situated in 20 acres at the end of the peninsula of Cap d'Antibes. Restaurant overlooking the Mediterranean, swimming pool, seaside cabanas, tennis, waterskiing, skin diving, private harbor.

Hotel Carlina, 73120 Courchevel. A very comfortable hotel at the base of the ski slopes near the lifts. Closed from April 24 to December 20.

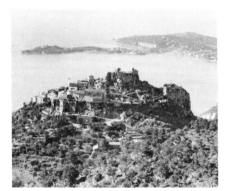

Cap Estel Hotel, Eze-Sur-Mer, France.

Pralong 2000, 73120 Courchevel. Good, modern hotel in the heart of ski country. Swimming pool, sauna. Closed April 15 to December 20.

Cap Estel Hotel, 06360 Eze-Bord-de-Mer. Formerly a princely residence, the Cap Estel was converted into a 45-room deluxe hotel in 1969. All rooms face the sea; superb cuisine served in a Louis XVI dining room or on the terrace; five-acre park, indoor and outdoor swimming pools, private beach, solarium.

Hotel Le Totem, 74300 Flaine. At the foot of 100 kilometers of ski trails, a fine modern hotel with old-fashioned comfort and innovative cuisine. Closed April 25 to July 7 and August 31 to December 27. Tennis and horseback riding in summer.

Chalet du Mont d'Arbois, 74120 le Mont d'Arbois, Route du Mont d'Arbois, Mégève. A peaceful mountain chalet at the foot of the ski slopes on the sunny side of Mont d'Arbois. Golf, tennis, horseback riding, swimming pool.

Hotel Negresco, 37, Promenade des Anglais, 06000 Nice. Designated a National Monument by the French government, magnificently located on the Promenade des Anglais facing the sea. Flowered terraces, private beach and garden. Gourmet restaurant with Gay Nineties atmosphere.

Mas de Serres, 06570 St.-Paul-de-Vence. A very private hideaway. Only six rooms with patios, big walled garden, excellent food. Ten minutes' drive from Fondation Maeght, one of the great museums of modern art.

Le Byblos, La Citadelle, 83990 St. Tropez. North African style with only 60 rooms and a glorious view of the Gulf of St. Tropez. Famous nightclub, Les Caves du Roy; heated swimming pool, solarium, waterskiing. Nearby: golf, tennis, horseback riding.

Hotel le Solaise, 73150 Val d'Isère. In one of the most fashionable ski areas, near the lifts. Fine cuisine, charming ambience. Golf and fishing nearby, Closed from April 18 to December 18.

Château Saint Martin, Route de Coursegoules, 06 Vence. (Also known as Domaine Saint Martin.) Castlelike, with a magnificent view of the seacoast from Nice to St. Raphael. Private terraces and balconies, villas, tennis, swimming pool. Renowned cuisine. Nearby: golf, horseback riding, water sports, fishing, skiing, mountain climbing.

Barge cruises, Floating Through Europe, 501 Madison Avenue, New York, New York 10022. A totally relaxed way to see the sun-drenched heart of France from her rivers. Whether drifting dreamily through the lush Burgundian countryside, redolent of ancient vineyards and gastronomic marvels, or

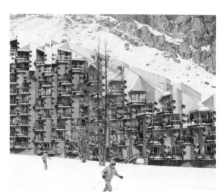

Val d'Isere, France.

the Mediterranean world of the Canal du Midi with whitewashed cottages and medieval towers gleaming in the southern sun, passengers will always find luxurious accommodations, fine food, and wine, interesting shore excursions. Floating Through Europe, Continental Waterways, and Wirreanda Cruises offer various arrangements, from accommodation on hotel boats to full charters.

GERMANY

"It subdues the impulse to work, one lives more casually, more humanly." That

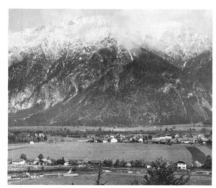

Bavarian Alps, Germany.

mental images that we all form, "There is a German Greece, a French Greece, and English Greece—there may even be an American one—all quite different." Very true, and there is also a vacationer's Greece, a sun-seeker's Greece, a Greece for the weary and dysphoric that soothes the body and lifts the spirit. One can relax on the beach in luxury on the outskirts of Athens or find total informality on small islands like Lemnos and Mykonos, where pleasant rooms for rent in private homes far outnumber traditional hotel rooms. Or seek very special places like gentle Corfu, with its strong Venetian and British influences, and rugged Crete, the proud repository of ancient Minoan civilization.

Grande Bretagne, Athens. Dominating Constitution Square in the center of the city, one of Europe's truly great hotels and an international meeting place. Classic cuisine, old-world service, luxurious base for sightseeing in and around Athens.

Elounda Beach Hotel, Aghios Nikolaos, Crete. Cretan-style bungalows on a beautiful beach overlooking the Gulf of Mirabello. Reputation for good food and service. Terrace restaurant. Swimming pool with bar, water sports, taverna, open-air theater and cinema.

Hotel Castello, Corfu. A Florentine-style castle, once the residence of King George II of Greece, now a luxury hotel in a 25-acre park. Large terrace overlooking the sea, open-air dining rooms and lounges. Private beach, water sports, tennis court. Eight miles from the town of Corfu.

Alkistis Hotel, San Stefano Beach, Mykonos. Ultramodern whitewashed bungalows with verandas on the beach. Restaurant, nightclub, waterskiing, sailing, canoeing, skin diving. Island has do-what-you-like atmosphere, all-night tavernas, nudist beaches, traditional family vacation spots.

Hotel Akti Myrina, Myrina, Lemnos. Deluxe bungalows on the beach in a scenic area. Swimming pool, two tennis courts, water sports, fishing. Otherwise, the island is poor in hotels but has picturesque villages with many small squares where the visitor can sit and sip a drink while watching the bustling activity of a very small world.

Astir Palace Hotel & Bungalows, Vouliagmeni Beach, Athens. An exclu-

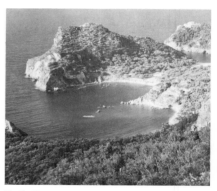

Corfu, Greece.

sive seaside resort on a 50-acre pine-clad promontory 15 miles from Athens along the Apollo Coast Highway. Two private beaches, indoor and outdoor swimming pools, sauna and health center, mini-golf, tennis, waterskiing, boating, yacht marina, championship golf course at Glyfada Beach Club nearby.

ITALY

Italy has beaches and ski resorts, pervasive reminders of antiquity and equally pervasive incursions of mind-boggling modernity. Practically everything has happened here at one time or another and the Italians have learned to take it all in their stride. They have been welcoming visitors for thousands of years—ancient Greeks, Christian pilgrims, English aristocrats on the Grand Tour, students, poets, jet-setters, package tourists—and they know how to do it with finesse and friendliness.

Hotel Villa Cipriani, 31011 Via Canova 298, Asolo. An exquisite house with only 32 rooms perched on a hillside overlooking the ancient town of Asolo. Eleanora Duse once lived here and so did Robert Browning. A peaceful place in a mild climate. Swimming and tennis nearby.

Grand Hotel Quisisana, Capri. Has been called the best hotel with the best swimming pool on the island. Lovely gardens, fine food and service, charming ambience.

Residence Punta Tragara, 80073 Capri. Romantic villa designed by Le Corbusier, overlooking the ocean. Each room is a suite with dining room and terrace. Landscaped saltwater pool, ther-

was once written about the sunniest part of Germany, in and around Lake Constance ("Bodensee" in German) with Italian blue skies and balmy temperatures. Actually *in* the lake are three enchanting small islands: Mainau, Reichenau, and Lindau.

On Mainau, Count Lennart Bernadotte, president of the German Gardening Society, lives in a castle amid subtropical vegetation. A special vacation package for women only includes being received at the castle by the Countess. Reichenau is known for its remarkable Romanesque churches built in the eighth to the tenth centuries. Lindau is an island city and port, free of cars and full of romantic byways and garden restaurants.

Steigenberger Inselhotel D-7750 Konstanz/Bodensee. A famous old hotel on a four-and-a-half-acre island just touching the city of Constance. The building, a thirteenth-century Dominican monastery, has modern comforts but retains its ancient beauty. Lake swimming and a motor yacht for cruises on Lake Constance. Nearby: mini-golf, tennis, windsurfing, sailing, waterskiing, fishing and rowing, horseback riding, gliding, clay pigeon shooting.

Hotel Bad Schachen, Lindau/Schachen. A palatial hotel in the grand manner on the banks of Lake Constance. Indoor and outdoor swimming pools, tennis, water sports, private beach. Nearby: golf, horseback riding. Closed from the end of October to the beginning of April.

GREECE

W. H. Auden once commented on the

mal baths, gourmet dining room, discotheque. No children or pets. Open from April to October.

Cristallo Palace Hotel, 32043 Cortina d'Ampezzo. An elegant turn-of-the-century building surrounded by seven acres of pine forest in one of Italy's most fashionable ski resorts. Hotel has distinguished reputation. Swimming pool, sauna, curling, ice skating, tennis courts, children's playrooms.

Hotel Pavillon, 11013 Courmayeur. A luxurious 40-room ski and summer resort at the foot of Mont Blanc. Indoor swimming pool, sauna and massage, golf nearby. Restaurant on the slopes in winter.

Hotel Regina Isabella, 80076 Lacco Ameno, Ischia. A deluxe hotel on the sea, connecting directly with the Regina Isabella and Santa Restituta Thermal Baths, which offer all types of thermal treatments. The radioactive mineral hot springs here have been famous since the seventh century B.C., but the present spa is completely modern. Hotel has indoor and outdoor thermal swimming pools, private beaches, water sports, tennis, mini-golf, bowling.

Grand Hotel & La Pace, 51016 Montecatini, Terme. Distinguished resort hotel and spa on private estate with park and flowering gardens in the middle of town near the thermal establishments. Masterful architecture, antique furnishings, no two rooms alike. Gourmet restaurant, dietetic restaurant with organic health food, open-air restaurant. Swimming pool, gymnasium, tennis court, complete spa facilities.

Hotel San Pietro, 84017 Positano. A picturesque 50-room hotel hewn from

Positano, Italy.

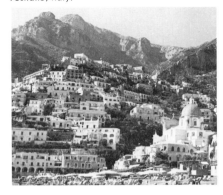

a cliff overlooking the loveliest part of the Amalfi coast. All rooms have terraces and floor-to-ceiling windows facing the sea, glass-walled marble bathrooms. Swimming pool, lawn tennis, and a private beach reachable only by elevator.

Hotel Rio Envers Gallia, 10054 San Sicario. An attractive ski resort in a sunny area of the Piedmont near Turin. Ski lifts a few yards from the hotel. Tennis, swimming nearby. Park of a 300-kilometer frontierless ski area between Italy and France. Closed April 1 to December 12.

Hotel Cala di Volpe, 07020 Porto Cervo, Sardinia. Charming isolated village-style resort directly on the Costa Smeralda. All rooms have terraces, breathtaking views, elegant traditional furnishings. Private harbor and beaches, tennis, and 18-hole golf course nearby. Open April to October.

Hotel Pitrizza, Porto Cervo 07020, Sardinia. Six stone villas scattered amid rocks and flowers, each with lounge, patio and four to eight bedrooms. Central club house has lounges, bar, restaurant. Beaches, swimming pool carved out of the rocks. Fine cuisine. Open May to October.

Hotel Principe di Piemonte, 10058 Sestriere. One of the few deluxe ski resorts in the Italian Alps. In a mountain valley, beautiful views. Sestriere facilities include 18 ski lifts, 100 kilometers of trails, hockey, curling, bowling, ski school, 30 restaurants, 11 nightclubs, two bars, two tearooms.

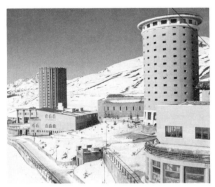

Sestriere, Italy.

San Domenico Palace Hotel, 98039 San Domenico, Taormina, Sicily. A sprawling fourteenth-century Dominican

monastery filled with antique treasures that has been a renowned hotel for almost a century. Spectacular gardens and grounds. Private beach, outdoor swimming pool, waterskiing, fishing, large gardens, exceptional view.

Hotel Cipriani, 30100 Venice, Giudecca 10. A palazzo beautifully situated on the lagoon with a view of the Lido. Private motor launch service around the clock to Piazza San Marco. Dining terrace overlooking Venetian gardens. Sea Gull Club with Olympic swimming pool, sunbathing facilities, and outdoor restaurant. Tennis courts, golf nearby. Names of famous guests never publicized.

Excelsior Palace Hotel, 30126 Venice, Lido. The hotel that made the Lido famous. Lavish decor. Fashionable private beach, all water sports, tennis, golf, horseback riding. Boat service to the mainland. Beach restaurant and bar, nightclub with rising floor. Open April to October.

Grand Hotel Des Bains, 30126 Venice, Lido. Gorgeous hotel connected with its private beach by underground passage. Startlingly Polynesian thatched-roof beach cabanas. Swimming pool, all water sports, tennis, golf, children's playgrounds. Rapid connections with Venice and the mainland.

MONACO

There's more in Monaco than Princess Grace. To see, there's the aquarium of the Musée Océanographique, the Jardin Exotique and the spectacular caverns of the Observatoire Grottos. To do, there's swimming (pools are best, the beaches are pebbly), skin diving, sailing, big game fishing, waterskiing, tennis, squash, bowling, and golfing. To watch, there's opera, concerts, ballet, football, fencing, boxing, gymnastics and, of course, the Monaco Grand Prix in May. At the famous Casino de Monte Carlo formal dress is required and the minimum age is twenty-one, but there are smaller nightclubs and discotheques where the atmosphere is more relaxed. The fashionable season is winter, when the climate is mild but definitely not warm.

Hotel de Paris, Place du Casino, Monte Carlo. An awesomely opulent *grande dame* opened in 1864, it overlooks the harbor and the Prince's palace. The wine cellar has 150,000 bottles and the Empire Room restaurant is a temple

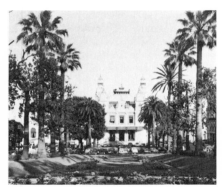

Casino Monte Carlo, Monaco.

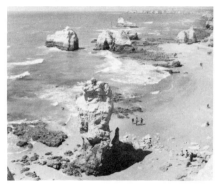

Algarve Coast, Portugal.

of gastronomy once presided over by Escoffier. There's an indoor seawater swimming pool, saunas and solaria. A guest card offers free access to the Casino, Monte Carlo beach, Monte Carlo Country Club with 20 tennis courts, Monte Carlo Golf Club, and Jimmy'z (sic) discotheque.

PORTUGAL

Political upheavals drove the tourists away for a while, but they're coming back now, and for good reason. It's a gentle, lovely country with gentle, peaceful people. A Portuguese, it is said, will raise his arm to strike a blow in anger, then smile sheepishly and lower it because he wouldn't dream of hurting anyone. And despite a fondness for bullfights, they don't kill the bull. Over 500 miles of golden beaches, white clouds of almond blossom in the Algarve in February, castles perched on craggy heights, the heady bite of *vinho verde* and the velvet caress of old port, more ways of cooking codfish than Boston ever dreamed of—that's Portugal for the visitor, and a very nice place it is.

Hotel Palacio, Estoril. A deluxe hotel in the resort favored by unemployed royalty, only 20 minutes from Lisbon. Fine service and cuisine. Gambling casino just across the garden from the hotel, outdoor swimming pool, tennis, guest privileges at Estoril Golf Club. Sauna and health baths nearby.

Penina Golf Hotel, Penina, Algarve. A large, grand hotel, excellent for year-round golf vacations. Eighteen-hole championship course, nine-hole course and practice course: all greens fees in-

cluded in room rate. Enormous swimming pool, tennis, horseback riding, bowling, croquet, transport to beach in summer.

Reid's Hotel, Estrada Monumental 139, Funchal, Madeira. A landmark hotel in acres of semitropical gardens on Portugal's "Garden Island." Perched on a cliff, the hotel has elevators that descend to sea level where there is a private bathing jetty and secluded sunbathing terraces. Two seawater swimming pools part-way down the cliff (reached by elevator), waterskiing, fishing, sailing, wind surfing, skin diving, tennis. Famous for its New Year's Eve party.

SCANDINAVIA

Scandinavia and skiing go together like herring and potatoes. It all started in Norway 4000 years ago when Stone Age man realized that sliding on snow was a lot easier than trying to walk through it. We know that because he left cave paintings of himself doing what is now called cross-country skiing or ski touring. Ski jumping was invented by Norwegian farmers jumping off the snow-laden roofs of their farmhouses. But Scandinavia has a summer face, too, warm and flowery and appreciated all the more because of its short duration.

Haikko Manor, 06400 Porvoo 40, Finland. One of Finland's best-known stately homes since 1362, the manor is now a distinguished 30-room country hotel with a magnificent view of the Gulf of Finland. It stands in 24 acres of green lawns with inviting walks and playing fields, overlooking a sandy beach with a log sauna. There's also an indoor swim-

ming pool with sauna. Adjacent to the hotel is the Haikko Health Spa, which offers many types of therapeutic baths, gymnastics and underwater massage and exercise. A six-pound weight loss in seven days is guaranteed.

Bardøla Høyfjellshotel, Geilo, Norway. An exceptionally comfortable modern hotel in Scandinavia's largest winter sports center. Preeminently ski touring country, but beginner and intermediate slopes for downhill skiers. Outdoor and indoor swimming pools, physical therapy room, gymnasium, sauna, solarium. In Geilo itself are nine ski lifts, the country's largest ski school, ice skating, curling, and facilities for renting all kinds of sporting equipment. At the Høyfjellshotel, as in most Norwegian country hotels, the smorgasbord breakfasts and lunches beggar description—superb salmon trout and a hundred other splendid dishes for Viking appetites.

Hotel Continental, Stortingsgaten 24126 Oslo, Norway. Traditional elegance in a convenient location between the Royal Palace and City Hall. Good restaurants, generous breakfast buffet. Ground-floor Theatercafeen is *the* meeting place of Oslo. Featherbeds and seven-foot-long bathtubs. Ski touring holidays in the city of Oslo are new and popular. Stay at the Continental in urban luxury and ski miles of trails in Holmenkollen and Frognesetter Parks.

Grand Hotel, Karl Johan Street, Oslo, Norway. Even more lavishly decorated in the grand manner than the Continental; otherwise, the same description fits. But the Grand must be singled out for its Bonanza restaurant: "A true American-Mexican restaurant with Western food, music and dancing." Why not?

Visby Hotel, Visby, Götland, Sweden. Bookings through Gotlandvesor AB, Box 81, S-621 of Visby. A modern 92-room hotel, the leading one in the city, portions of which are in a medieval building. Visby has existed since the Stone Age and reached its climax of wealth and power at the end of the thirteenth century. It's a fascinating medieval city, ideal for walking and exploring, has many good restaurants serving saffron pancakes and other Götland specialties. Visby is the only city on the island of Götland in the Baltic Sea, less than 3000 square miles in area but rich in history and stringently preserved as a memento of

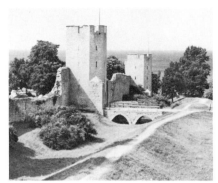
Visby, Gotland Island, Sweden.

old Sweden. Beautiful beaches, bird sanctuary, open-air museum. Summer festivals of medieval pageantry and Viking sporting events.

SPAIN

It has been said that Europe ends at the Pyrenees, and, indeed, great chunks of European experience seem to have completely bypassed Spain. However, post-Franco relaxation has led to far greater receptivity to (although not necessarily acceptance of) modern European and even American tastes and customs. Tourism is booming, and, while some of the projects seem ill-conceived and inimical to the very things that inspire people to come to Spain in the first place, there are some shining examples of creative innovation as well as of lovingly maintained tradition. Wherever you go in Spain, remember that dinner is never served before 9:30—and that's for earlybirds—and men and women dress conservatively at all times.

Parador Nacional "San Francisco," Granada. Picturesque and charming, high on a hill in the very walls of the Moorish Alhambra, restrained Spanish decor with museum-quality woodcarving, terraces overlooking the city and the gardens of the Alhambra. Try to reserve a year in advance.

Hotel Los Monteros, Marbella, Costa del Sol. Country club ambience in modern buildings incorporating the best in traditional Spanish design. Tennis club with ten courts and five squash courts (Lew Hoad is resident pro and manager), indoor and outdoor swimming pools, Riding Club, 18-hole golf course,

gymnasium, saunas, Cabana Club on the beach. Beautiful location.

Marbella Club Hotel, Marbella, Costa del Sol. Andalucian-styled bungalows and suites in a subtropical garden surrounded by 11 championship golf courses. Beach with straw-roofed huts, two swimming pools, paddle tennis, waterskiing, boating, windsurfing, sauna.

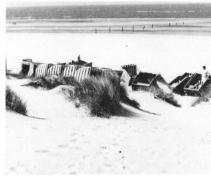
Baltic Coast.

Hotel Son Vida, Palma de Mallorca. A thirteenth-century castle now a lavish hotel besieged by celebrities. Esther Williams swam here, Brigitte Bardot sunbathed; Aristotle Onassis, most of the Eisenhowers and Nixons, Princess Grace, the Maharanee of Baroda, and Eben Whittlesey, the mayor of Carmel, California, have at various times disported themselves in its 1400 acres of subtropical park. Swimming pool, tennis, golf, horseback riding.

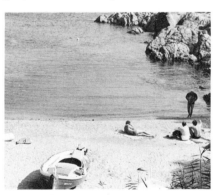
S'Agaro, Costa Brava, Spain.

Hostal de la Gavina, S'Agaro, Costa Brava. An ancient Catalan palace on a Mediterranean peninsula between two

beaches. Rooms furnished in styles of various epochs and regions of Spain, no two alike. Red and black marble baths, four-poster beds. Award-winning cuisine. Swimming pool, sauna, tennis, gymnasium. Nearby: 18-hole golf course, riding stables, and yacht harbor.

Sotogrande Hotel, Apartado 1. Sotogrande, Cadiz. Part of a deluxe hotel, golf club and private villa development on 4200 acres at one of the Costa del Sol's finest beaches, 12 miles from Gibraltar. Two Robert Trent Jones-designed golf courses, six tennis courts, horseback riding, trap and skeet shooting, polo, fronton, four swimming pools.

Parador Nacional "Conde de Orgaz," Toledo. The best way to experience Toledo (merely to see it is not enough) is to stay there at least overnight and this is the best place to stay. Old and atmospheric, distinguished and comfortable. The view from its balconies gives one the feeling of being inside an El Greco painting.

SWITZERLAND

The tourist industry in Switzerland is something like brain surgery in other countries. It's not a field for amateurs who think it might be fun. Rather, it's a dedicated profession whose practitioners are educated, trained, inspected, and certified. Anywhere in the world, "Swiss management" in a hotel's advertising is a phrase that brings joy to the heart of the harried traveler, secure in the knowledge that he will be well taken care of.

Bellevue Palace, 5 Kochergasse, Berne. Official residence of visiting dignitaries, next to the Parliament building and close to all shopping. Magnificent view of the Bernese Alps, skiing within minutes of the hotel. In winter, curling and skating; in summer, golf, riding, fishing, shooting, boating, and tennis.

Grand Hotel Regina, 3818 Grindelwald. One of the most complete summer and winter resort hotels in the Alps. All winter sports, cozy fireplaces. Hiking, mountaineering, indoor and outdoor swimming pools, tennis. Golf nearby. Open December 15 to October 15.

Palace Hotel, 3780 Gstaad. Deluxe ski and summer resort, adjacent to 30 ski lifts and cable cars. Slopes for all grades of skiers. Skiing on Diablerets Glacier all year. Skating, curling, tobogganing,

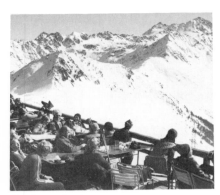

Alps, Switzerland.

riding, hiking, indoor and outdoor swimming pools, golf, trout fishing, bowling, tennis, skeet and trap shooting. Open December 10 to March 30 and June to September.

Palace Hotel, St. Moritz. One of the world's most luxurious hotels, on the lake in the center of town, near ski areas. International society clientele. French cuisine, special diets, produce from hotel's own farm. Private staff of ski guides, indoor swimming pool, ice skating, curling, bobsledding, helicopter service for skiers. In summer, riding school, clay-pigeon shooting, mountaineering, gliding, yachting, trout fishing, tennis, summer skiing.

Mont Cervin-Seilerhaus, 3920 Zermatt. Good traditional hotel with indoor swimming pool. Zermatt, at the foot of the Matterhorn, is free of automobiles and accessible only by train. It has the longest ski season in the Alps. Activities

available: curling, skating, hockey, ski and mountaineering school, Alpine and cross-country skiing. Open end of November to beginning of April and end of June to mid-October.

YUGOSLAVIA

Ten years ago, Yugoslavia was a destination for the knowing few, those who were willing to endure some inconveniences for the reward of enjoying the natural beauty, fascinating historical landmarks, friendly people and delicious food of this most Westernized of Balkan countries. Nowadays Yugoslavia is not only "in," it's popular because more and more people have become aware of such delights as Bled's balmy summer climate and fine winter skiing, Dubrovnik's perfectly preserved medieval beauty, and Sveti Stefan's brilliant transformation from a fishing village into a luxury hotel. Along the sunny Dalmatian Coast, it's warm enough for sea swimming until early November.

Grand Hotel Toplice, Bled. Grandly Old World on a magnificent site on the shores of Lake Bled, with views of the lake, ancient castle, and Julian Alps. Healthy subalpine climate, longest bathing season of all Alpine resorts. Swimming pool fed by a thermal spring, sauna and massage, solarium and gymnasium, lake beach and boating. Tennis and golf nearby. Bled is eight kilometers from a newly developed ski area, which boasts of skiing from November to May. Other winter activities are ice skating, ski touring, sledging, and curling.

Dubrovnik Palace Hotel, Dubrov-

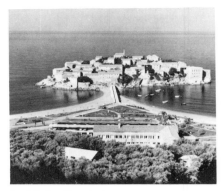

Sveti Stefan, Yugoslavia.

nik. Beautifuly located next to the ancient city walls on the tip of Dubrovnik's peninsula jutting into the Adriatic sea. Private bathing beach, swimming pool, swimming season May to October. All of Dubrovnik is a perfectly preserved—but *living*—museum, with no automobiles allowed within the walled city.

Hotel Sveti Stefan, Sveti Stefan. An entire island fishing village, fortified more than 500 years ago against Turkish pirates and buccaneers, converted into a luxury hotel, the showpiece of the Yugoslav tourist industry. There are 133 suites, each an old cottage or house renovated for comfort but retaining its charm. The island is a small jewel, with little squares, cobblestoned streets, and old churches. Two fine private beaches, one with a terrace restaurant under the olive trees, facing the sunset. There's also a swimming pool hewn from the rocks and a casino.

17. Africa and the Near East

EGYPT

Egypt has cachet as well as endless history embodied in such monuments and places as the Pyramids, the Valley of the Kings, the great Temple at Karnak, the Colossi of Memnon, and the tomb of King Tutankhamun. Hotel space is short, so always have firm reservations. The native cuisine is delicious and imaginative, and the belly dancing is declared by those who know the best in the Middle East.

Isis and Osiris Floating Hotels, Aswan to Luxor. Write c/o Nile Hilton, Takrir Square, Cairo, Egypt. Operated by Hilton International, these 48-cabin cruisers are the most luxurious on the Nile, with swimming pool and sun deck, air conditioning, shore excursions with qualified guides. Itinerary covers Egypt's most spectacular antiquities. Casual clothing in daytime, jacket and tie at night. Temperatures over 100 degrees from June to September but cooler in the evening.

IVORY COAST

The capital, Abidjan, is a boom town,

prosperous and growing in all directions. But there's also the interior—true jungle with fascinating villages and indigenous cultures. If arranging a tour presents difficulties, bear with it—remember that tourism has not yet developed much beyond the coast and that outside the big hotels French is the only European language spoken.

Hotel Ivoire Inter-Continental, Boulevard de la Comiches (P.O. Box 8001), Abidjan. In one of the fastest growing and most modern cities in Africa, the Ivoire is a 30-story gleaming white fantasy on the shore of Ebrie Lagoon with landscaped gardens and reflecting pools. Fully air conditioned, swimming pool with bar, artificial lake, water sports, tennis, bowling, golf, sauna and massage, gymnasium, heliport and—would you believe?—ice skating rink!

KENYA

Nothing can match a safari where you see elephants, giraffes, zebras, and dozens of other wild creatures in their natural environment, so close you could—but won't—touch them. Kenya has lovely beaches at Mombasa and lively city life

in Nairobi, but seeing the animals is the overriding reason for coming here.

Salt Lick-Taita Hills Game Lodges, Taita Hills, Bura. Correspondence c/o Nairobi Hilton, P.O. Box 30624, Nairobi, Kenya. Small, exclusive lodges operated by Hilton International with club atmosphere and fine restaurants located between the east and west sections of Tsavo National Park, Kenya's largest game reserve. Taita Hills, with swimming pool, bird walks, and gardens, serves as a base lodge for exploring the park. Salt Lick, six miles away, offers close-up viewing of animals from luxurious thatched-roof rondavel cottages on stilts over salt lick water holes. Casual dress at both places; for safaris wear neutral-colored clothing with long sleeves, sturdy shoes, sun hat, and scarf or mask for dust protection.

MOROCCO

Morocco has a small piece of the Sahara Desert, it's true, but it also has forests, lakes, the snowy Atlas Mountains and endless coastal beaches on both the Mediterranean and the Atlantic. It's a growing destination for tourists and a good one, with a wide range of sporting activities, fine French and native cuisine, and an astonishing variety of quality goods to buy.

Club Méditerranée, Marrakesh. Bookings through travel agents or American Express. One of Club Med's most lavish year-round resort villages, resembling an ancient Arab town with floating gardens and shaded arcades. White stuccoed bedrooms with sitting area and Moorish-style sunken circular bathtubs. Air conditioned throughout. Outdoor swimming pool, Turkish bath, gymnasium, yoga, volley ball, golf nearby shuttle service to "The Palmeraie," the Club's 1,000-acre annex village on the outskirts of Marrakesh, with swimming pool, Arabian horses, tennis, archery, pitch and putt golf.

La Mamounia Hotel, Avenue Boub Jdid, Marrakesh. Deluxe hotel in garden within the Old City walls. Fully air conditioned, balconied rooms overlooking Atlas Mountains and orange gardens. Swimming pool with sun deck, sauna, Turkish bath. Churchill's favorite.

Malabata Hotel, Tangier. The only deluxe hotel in Tangier directly on its own private beach. Fully air conditioned, balconies, several restaurants and lounges. Swimming pool, water sports, mini-golf, tennis, volley ball.

SENEGAL

Dakar has such a romantic reputation that one is apt to forget that it's in a country called Senegal, which is full of nonurban attractions. Despite the long-standing drought, the country has made heroic efforts to preserve its wildlife. The most important visitable game parks are Niokolo-Koba, rich in landscapes and the folklore of its many ethnic groups; Djoudj Bird Reserve, one of the most ancient areas of European colonization; and Basse Camance, famous for the many species of monkeys who live in its forests of tropical trees.

Club Méditerranée, Les Almadies, Dakar. Bookings through travel agents or American Express. Three-storied Moorish-style air-conditioned hotel on a 71-acre landscaped oceanfront estate on the Cape Verde Peninsula. Huge swimming pool as well as ocean swimming, eight floodlit tennis courts, sailing, yoga, calisthenics, volley ball, deep-sea fishing. Interesting excursions available. Summers

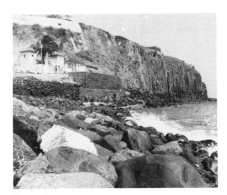
Senegal.

hot and breezy; winters warm during the day with cool mornings and evenings.

Hotels Méridien, Boite Postale 8092, Dakar-Yoff. A complex of three hotels—the Diarama, N'Gor and Village N'Gor—on the tip of the Cape Verde Peninsula, protected from ocean storms by a barrier reef. The Diarama and N'Gor are modern, low-rise hotels; the Village N'Gor is composed of individual thatched-roof bungalows in a 25-acre tropical park. Guests share sports, restaurant and entertainment facilities of all three hotels. Private beach, two swimming pools, tennis, horseback riding, volley ball, sailing, deep-sea fishing.

SOUTH AFRICA

Probably the most beautiful country in the world, South Africa is a nature-lover's paradise with incredible variety in its animals and vegetation, miles of beaches for swimming and surfing and the best game conservation program on the continent. Hotels are generally excellent and the food is good. The "braai," or barbecue, is a national specialty, as are Afrikaaner dishes like *bobotie* and *sosaties.* Dress is always conservative but quite sophisticated in the cities.

Alphen Hotel, P.O. Box 35, Alphen Drive, 7848 Constantia, Cape Town. One of South Africa's most beautiful hotels. Dating from 1750, it's an exquisite example of Cape Dutch architecture—a simplified country version of European Baroque—and the property is still a producing wine farm. Swimming pool; tennis nearby. Golf, horseback riding, and beach ten minutes away. A comfortable base for touring the beautiful and historic Cape Peninsula.

The President Hotel, Beach Road (Box 62), Sea Point, Cape Town. Traditional colonial-style top-class hotel in manicured gardens not far from the central areas of Cape Town and near the municipal golf course. Swimming pool, afternoon tea in the garden, spacious rooms.

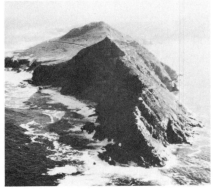
Cape Point, South Africa.

Cabana Beach Hotel, Lagoon Drive (Box 10), Umhlanga Rocks, Natal. On the Indian Ocean near the resort city of Durban, a stunning modern hotel with furnishings one yearns to take home. Beach, swimming pool, water sports. Several restaurants, excellent food, Zulu dancing.

MalaMala Game Reserve, P.O. Box 3741, Durban 4000, Transvaal. The ultimate outdoor experience—a luxurious, private, 50,000-acre game reserve and top-flight resort on the edge of Kruger National Park. One of the few places where you can go on individual safari on foot or in Land Rover with a personal guide. Accommodations in air-conditioned thatched huts, gourmet cuisine with wine, swimming pool, room service. Rates include laundry and afternoon tea. Informal dress. Best season for game viewing, late May to late September. Although the weather is sunny all year round, remember that the seasons are reversed and the hot summer is from October to April.

TUNISIA

This is the place to see the best-preserved Roman remains in the world as well as examples of a dazzling Islamic heritage, not only in the holy city of Kairouan—second only to Mecca—but also in the

172

labyrinthine medinas of Sousse and Tunis, with their bustling souks and ancient mosques. The major resort centers are Hammamet, Sousse, Monastir, and the island of Djerba where the climate is hot and dry the year round even though it gets cold in the interior in winter.

Hotel Dar Djerba (also spelled Jerba), Ile de Djerba. The third largest hotel in the world, with 2500 rooms divided into four classes of accommodations. All are in North African-styled attached bungalows, but the deluxe version consists of spacious air conditioned duplexes with drawing room, bedroom, bathroom, two lavatories, refrigerator, two radios, two telephones, balcony and view over the garden to the sea. There's also a separate children's hotel for ages six to twelve with counselors, plus nursery and kindergarten for daytime or overnight stays. Discotheque, nightclub, casino, horseback riding, Arab marketplace, pizzeria, three swimming pools (one Olympic size, one thermal), children's pool, beautiful beach, tennis, sailing, underwater fishing, camelback riding on the beach, volleyball, Ping-Pong, bowling. Despite all the activities available, the atmosphere is one of simple elegance, privacy and spaciousness.

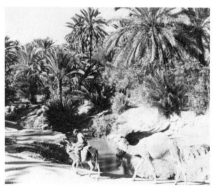

Djerba, Tunisia.

IRAN

Tehran may once have been a beautiful city and it may be so once again someday, but for the time being it's a place to get out of fast and go on to Shiraz, Persepolis, and the Caspian Coast in order to see the beauty and sense the atmosphere of ancient Persia and modern Iran.

Hyatt Regency Caspian, P.O. Box 99, Chalus, Manakabrood. Palatial enough to hold its own among the princely properties of the titled and the famous that line the Caspian Coast. On the site of an ancient tea plantation, the hotel is characterized by boldly dramatic modern design and decoration. Huge outdoor swimming pool with swim-up bar and cabanas. Balconied rooms, casino, caviar bar.

Hyatt Omar Khayyam, P.O. Box 182, Farah Avenue, Mashhad. A contemporary echo of a Persian palace surrounded by a private park in an ancient city of mosques and shrines. Sumptuously furnished rooms with Persian miniatures and artifacts, restaurants and supper club with Iranian gourmet cuisine, dancing and entertainment. Outdoor swimming pool.

ISRAEL

When tourists started coming to modern Israel it was for religious pilgrimages or for sightseeing among the relics of antiquity. But now many people come for rest and relaxation in the fine resort hotels or the simple but comfortable kibbutz guest houses. Many come to the health spas built on the sites of mineral springs famous since biblical times for their curative properties.

Dan Caesarea Golf Hotel, Caesarea. Reservations Office: 99 Hayarkon Street, Tel Aviv. A beautiful hotel built by Baron de Rothschild overlooking the sea. It's a convenient base for touring the entire country and has the only 18-hole golf course in Israel. Swimming pool, tennis, horseback riding, skin diving, sailing, sauna, children's playground.

Laromme Eilat Hotel, P.O. Box 555, Eilat. A modern luxury hotel at the gateway to the Sinai Desert, Mount Sinai, King Solomon's Mines, Santa Katarina Monastery. Year-round sunshine and healthy desert climate. Beach, enormous saltwater swimming pool with swim-up snack bar, health club, sauna. Nearby: skin diving, sailing, waterskiing, glass-bottom boat rides.

Accadia Grand Hotel, P.O. Box 3300, Herzlia on Sea. On Israel's Riviera, a fashionable hotel in a country club setting only eight miles from Tel Aviv. Ocean swimming, swimming pool, sauna, tennis courts.

The Rimon Inn, Safed. High in the mountains of the Galilee, a medieval stone building transformed into a low-key luxury inn near the artists' quarter of Safed, an ancient center of Jewish mysticism. Fine cuisine and friendly service, swimming pool, terraced gardens.

TURKEY

The Middle East's best-kept secret—a huge, beautiful, intriguing country with spectacular scenery, good beaches, friendly people, superb food, and more Greek ruins than Greece itself. Tourism is still in the early stages, so that idyllic coastal areas like the Turquoise Coast don't have enough good hotels yet. Izmir is rather well-developed touristically because the French discovered its charms a long time ago. Istanbul is a disappointment at first glance, a knockout at second. Best hotels are the Hilton, Sheraton, and Inter-Continental, all with splendid views of the Bosphorus and the Golden Horn. In fact, each is probably among the best in its own chain—and an international-class chain hotel is a godsend in a developing country.

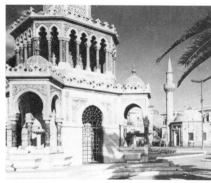

Izmir, Turkey.

Büyük Efes Oteli, Cumhüriyet Meydani, Izmir. Apart from the international chains, this is probably the best hotel in Turkey. Sweetly old fashioned, with lots of space, huge public rooms, large garden, outdoor swimming pool. Izmir is a delight, with its picturesque waterfront promenade reminiscent of the Croisette in Cannes. Friendly outdoor cafes where the water pipe is passed around. As in most of Turkey, remarkably good food—simple, subtle, and pleasing to all tastes.

18. Southeast Asia and the Pacific

AUSTRALIA

The best reason for going to Australia is to cuddle a koala bear. The next best reason is to see the Great Barrier Reef, which spreads for more than 1000 miles along the sunny coast of Queensland. Slowly built up over millions of years into a spectacular showcase of the sea, the reef is a series of coral banks separated by tortuous channels shading off from delicate green to the deepest blue. Great shoals of brilliantly colored fish glide through the coral gardens. Visitors can don snorkel and goggles to become part of this underwater world in the safety of a reef lagoon.

The Reef House, Palm Cove, North Queensland 4871. An ideal base for excursions to the Great Barrier Reef. Only 18 guests at a time can be lodged in this exclusive beachfront resort owned by a retired brigadier general and his wife. There's a friendly house party atmosphere with an honor system bar, Extensive wine cellar with good Australian vintages, tropical gardens, a mile of sand beach, trips to the Great Barrier Reef, snorkeling, game fishing.

BALI (INDONESIA)

Now that the rest of the world is going topless, Balinese girls are modestly covered. However, Bali's other beauties are still evident—miles of sugar-white beaches, softly swaying palm trees, lush green countryside filled with vibrantly colored flowers, jewel-box temples, and exquisite young dancers. Everything in Balinese life has religious significance, including tooth-filings and cremations,

Bali.

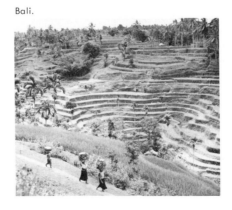

major events that are open to visitors. They are *cheerful* occasions, so don't pass them up!

Bali Hyatt, Sanur-Denpasar. Flamboyantly beautiful, right on the beach in one of the world's last paradises. Lobby has no walls. All rooms have balcony, air conditioning, tasteful Balinese decor. Swimming pool with swim-up bar, outdoor dining terrace, open-air theater for Balinese music and dance performances.

Bali Oberoi Hotel, P.O. Box 351, Denpasar. Thatched cottage villas and lanai suites furnished with Balinese works of art, air conditioned, a garden in each bathroom. Each villa or suite has its own team of houseboys, summoned by striking a gong. Mile-long private beach; scuba diving and surfing; the largest swimming pool in Bali; tennis and mini-golf; motor bikes, beach buggies, and horse carts for hire. Outdoor theater for Balinese dancing.

HAWAII

In these mid-Pacific islands East and West meet in a delightful stew of American efficiency, Chinese enterprise, Japanese diligence, and Polynesian *dolce far niente*. Everyone has thrown something into the pot, and the various flavors have rubbed off on one another while the ingredients have retained their own identities. Somehow it works, and the result—despite the urban overkill of Honolulu—is a tropical paradise with perfect plumbing, safe food and water, honest cab drivers, and a culturally diverse but harmonious population.

Kona Village Resort, P.O. Box 1299, Kaupulehu, Kailua-Kona, 96740. Seventy-one *hales* (thatched-roof bungalows) standing on stilts beside the beach or on a garden form a Polynesian village like those of old Hawaii and other Pacific islands—with all modern conveniences. Kona Village is best-known for its weddings—bride and groom come with or without friends and family (other guests love to attend the ceremonies) and the resort provides everything, including a minister. Besides getting married, activities include ocean and pool swimming, tennis, sailing, snorkeling, fishing, scuba diving, nature walks.

Mauna Kea Beach Hotel, Kamuela, 96743. Gently understated luxury characterizes this 310-room hotel set next to a curving beach on the Big Island of Hawaii. Guests are surrounded by superb works of oriental art, flowering courtyards, and graceful open terraces. Cuisine is international, supplemented by traditional Hawaiian luaus. Robert Trent Jones-designed golf course, riding and hunting on the famous Parker Ranch, nine tennis courts, swimming pool, sailing, deep-sea fishing, scuba diving, snorkeling, catamaran cruising.

Hotel Hana-Maui, Hana, Maui, 96713. A relaxed gathering of garden cottages surrounded by cascading waterfalls, tropical forest and a gentle sea on the very site where King Kamehameha I saw the first sailing ships to reach the islands and met Captain Cook and Captain Bligh. In addition to the beaches, there's a freshwater swimming pool, pitch-and-putt golf, horseback riding, tennis, surfing, night spear fishing, snorkeling, bicycle riding.

Kapalua Bay Hotel, P.O. Bin 188, Maui, 96732. Rockresorts' newest and most superb foray into elegant tropical living is contained in a series of low-profile interconnected buildings that

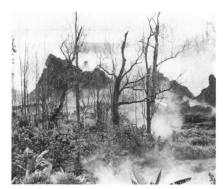
Hawaii Volcanoes National Park, Hawaii.

slope gently down to a white sand beach protected by a coral reef. Spacious rooms have separate living and sleeping areas, his-and-her bath areas, refrigerators, air conditioning and ceiling fans. Swimming pool with bar, ten tennis courts in a garden, 18-hole Arnold Palmer-designed championship golf course, international boutiques. Casual elegance is the style in the evenings; jackets are worn, ties are optional.

Kahala Hilton, 5000 Kahala Avenue, Honolulu, 96816. This is the secret Hilton, the connoisseurs' favorite, unpublicized, and nearly always full. Highrise but not too high, on an 800-foot expanse of golden sand beach with Diamond Head in the background. Sailing, surfing, snorkeling, swimming pool, catamaran sailing, deep-sea fishing, scuba diving. Orchids on your pillow at night.

HONG KONG

In Hong Kong the people are Chinese, the language is English, and the pace is frantic. One of the world's most exciting cities, it has an incomparable setting on a generous harbor backed by rugged green mountains. Climate is semitropical with rainy season in the summer; beautiful, balmy weather in spring and fall. There are two parts to the city: Hong Kong Island, where the original British settlement was established, and Kowloon, on the Chinese mainland. Both sections are well-supplied with fine hotels, marvelous restaurants, and the incredible variety of shops for which the city is famous. On Kowloon side, the traditional Peninsula, scene of Hong Kong's surrender to the Japanese and return to the

British in World War II, is the reigning hotel. Supreme on Hong Kong island is The Mandarin, the outside office-building modern, but the interior richly appointed and sybaritic.

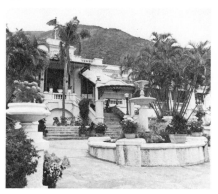
Repulse Bay Hotel, Hong Kong.

The Repulse Bay Hotel, Repulse Bay. Sister to The Peninsula, this gracious vestige of Colonial days lies on a palm-fringed vantage point overlooking Repulse Bay and one of Hong Kong's most beautiful beaches. The height of elegance in 1920 when it opened, it has been restored and refurbished to look as good as old. Spacious, high-ceilinged rooms, open-air Verandah Restaurant, buffet lunch served all afternoon. Visiting royalty and heads of state often stay here.

INDIA

India isn't a country, it's a subcontinent —enormous, varied, complex, dazzling. It overwhelms, entrances, shocks, mystifies. The past is ever-present, especially in places like Jaipur and Udaipur in the land of the Rajahs. But modern India is equally compelling, with bustling cities like Bombay, languorous beach resorts like Madras, and odd corners like Goa, now Indian but still Portuguese in atmosphere. Shop in India for splendid things—gold, jewels, silks, carved ivory, antique paintings, and sculptures.

The Taj Mahal Hotel and the Taj Inter-Continental, Apollo Bunder, 400039 Bombay. The 70-year-old traditional Taj Mahal lost none of its character or ambience in its recent merger with the high-rise Inter-Continental next door. Both are fine hotels, dominating Bom-

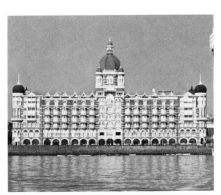

The Taj Intercontinental, Bombay, India.

bay's harbor at the Gateway of India. They can arrange golf and yachting for guests and they have a pier for sailboats. Round outdoor swimming pool, health clubs for men and women, gymnasium, yoga. Taj Mahal shops are best places in Bombay for luxury items.

Hotel Oberoi Bogmalo Beach, Bogmalo, Goa. Brand-new resort on a private beach in tranquil surroundings, owned by India's premiere hotel corporation. Air-conditioned rooms, outdoor swimming pool with sunken bar, restaurant overlooking the Arabian Sea, health club with sauna and massage.

The Fort Aguada Beach Resort, Sinquerim, Bardez, Goa. A tropical delight on the Arabian Sea, thought by many to be the best hotel in India. Air-conditioned rooms overlook the sea. There's a poolside bar and hammocks under the palm trees. Miles and miles of uncrowded beaches; pleasant, dry climate with constant breezes except for monsoon season June through September. Swimming pool, waterskiing, yachting, salmon and mackerel fishing, clay pigeon-shooting. Excellent fresh fish and lobster.

The Rambagh Palace Hotel, Bhawani Singh Road, Jaipur 5. Traditionally a residence of the royal family of Jaipur and a hotel since 1958, the Rambagh Palace is surrounded by majestic lawns and gardens only a ten-minute drive from the hub of the city and its fabulous bazaar. All 80 vast, cool rooms are furnished in palatial Rajasthani style. Swimming pool, tennis, squash, golf, shopping arcade. Indian and continental cuisine.

The Fisherman's Cove Beach Resort, Covelong Beach, Tamil Nadu, Madras. In the south of India on a sweeping crescent beach, artistically landscaped to blend in with the natural beauty and seclusion of Covelong Bay. Swimming pool, rowing, sailing, scuba diving. Convenient for excursions to Madras, Mahabalipuram, Kanchipuram, and Pondicherry.

The Lake Palace Hotel, Pichola Lake, Udaipur. A marble dream set in the blue waters of the Pichola Lake, the hotel appears to float in white marble splendor, a perfect blend of eighteenth-century elegance and twentieth-century luxury. All rooms overlook the lake and are furnished with the Maharana of Udaipur's personal heirlooms. Among other glories, it has a suite called "The Abode of Joy." Even the swimming pool is marble. There's also rowing, sailing, and fishing in the lake.

MACAO

Macao is a tiny Portuguese enclave on the Chinese mainland 40 miles from Hong Kong, sharing the same balmy climate. Hong Kong's Chinese love to go there to gamble in the sumptuous casinos. But it's also a delightful side-trip for visitors to Hong Kong, only 45 minutes away by jetfoil, 75 minutes by hydrofoil, or 2½ hours on restful steamers with cabins and restaurants. Food is good—both Chinese and Portuguese—and shopping bargains, especially in gold jewelry, are reputed to surpass Hong Kong's.

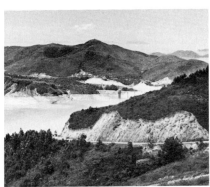

Lantau, Macao.

Bela Vista Hotel, Rua Comendador Kou Ho Neng. A grand old hotel with a history of more than a century of Portuguese hospitality. Soothingly peaceful, superb views. Restaurant, bar, terrace cafe. Strictly for unwinding.

Lisboa Hotel-Casino. Avenida da Amizade. One of the most lavish and extravagant hotels anywhere. A city within a city, with nightclubs, restaurants and bars, two-story-high casino, and shopping arcade. The architecture is wildly imaginative. Swimming pool, bowling, sauna, and steam baths.

Pousada de Coloane, Praia de Cheoc Van, Coloane Island. The Lisboa's peaceful annex, a place to get away from it all. Set in a pine forest overlooking a fine swimming beach. Only twelve rooms now, more to be built.

PHILIPPINES

Political upheaval and violence have in recent years characterized this 1200-mile chain of incredibly beautiful volcanic islands, but now—whatever one's opinion of the regime may be—travelers report that the country is calm and safe everywhere except for a few very remote areas and that visitors are warmly welcomed. The islands are rich in historical lore, the cuisine is tasty and varied, the hotels are good. Shopping highlights in addition to native handicrafts are pearl and coral jewelry, couturier women's fashions and internationally renowned cigars. The musicians and dancers are the best in Asia.

Punta Baluarte Inter-Continental, Calatagan, Bantangas, Bantangas City, 4001. A luxurious but cozy resort by the sea with well-appointed thatched-roof cottages nestled against the verdant hills. Swimming pools, tennis, pelota, line fishing, spear fishing, scuba diving, waterskiing, snorkeling, horseback riding, polo, Robert Trent Jones championship golf course.

Pagsanjan Rapids Hotel, Pagsanjan, Laguna. A comfortable, four-story resort built on the banks of the Pagsanjan River, close enough to Manila for day trips. Shooting mountain river rapids is the big attraction here. Swimming pool, billiards, table tennis.

Nalinac Beach Resort, Baguio, Luzon. On the calm waters of the South China Sea in a lush tropical setting about five hours' drive from Manila. Palm trees line deserted white beaches. Swimming pool, putting greens, boating, waterskiing, snorkeling, fishing.

Resort Pines, Baguio, Luzon. In com-

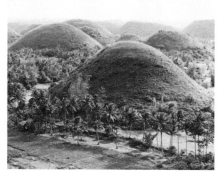

Chocolate Hills, Philippines.

fortable colonial style, it's considered one of the premiere hotels in the Philippines. The cool mountain town of Baguio is the most popular resort area in the islands. Tennis, pelota, swimming pool, sauna.

SRI LANKA

Sri Lanka—the Resplendent Isle—has been given many names over the years. It was called Taprobane by Greeks and Romans, Serendib by the Arabs, Ceilao by the Portuguese, Ceylan by the Dutch, and Ceylon by the British. By any name, it's a captivating little island with miles of golden beach edging coastal villages, acres of coconuts surrounding Buddhist temples, ruins of an ancient civilization lying in wooded parks and cool glades, peaceful game sanctuaries and richly forested mountains. Shopping is wonderful, especially for gold, silver, antiques, and handicrafts.

Bentota National Holiday Resort, Bentota. Three luxury hotels with 150 rooms in a resort complex of shops, cafeteria, open-air theater, fair grounds, art gallery, information center, and railway station on the site of an old Portuguese fort. Long stretch of sugar-white sand beach at the meeting-place of sea and river. Good base for touring the southern part of the country.

TAHITI

Everyone's dream spot, away from everywhere, on the way to nowhere. In other words, you don't get Tahiti as a stopover on many airline tickets, so maybe that's

the reason visitors tend to be wealthy and elderly. Tahiti and the other islands of French Polynesia—Les Iles Sous le Vent—are more beautiful than they look in the movies, and the romantic atmosphere is unsurpassed anywhere in the world. The major activity is unquestionably simply to enjoy life.

Hotel Bora Bora, Nunve, Bora Bora. Fifteen over-water bungalows with glass floor panels for observing tropical fish, also beach and garden bungalows. Scenic restaurant with fine food, beautiful white sand beaches. Tahitian *tamaaraas* (barbecues), all water sports.

Hotel Aimeo, Moorea. Mail to P.O. Box 627, Papeete. The only hotel in Moorea on gorgeous Cook's Bay. Over-water bungalows and beach bungalows. Tahitian entertainment and barbecues, boutique, perfect swimming in front of the hotel, fishing, outrigger canoe trips, bicycles.

Bali Hai, Moorea. Mail to P.O. Box 415, Papeete. Owned by three American drop-outs from the rat race, this was the first resort to build over-water bungalows with glass floor panels for fish-watching. White sand beach, open-air restaurant, Tahitian barbecues. Private swimming dock, tennis, all water sports. There are smaller Bali Hai hotels on the charming little islands of Raiatea and Huahine.

Moorea Lagon, Moorea. Mail to P.O. Box, 1660, Papeete. Forty-five beach and garden bungalows at the foot of Mount Rotui between Cook's Bay and Opunohu Bay. Beach restaurant. Beautiful white sand beach, swimming pool, water sports.

Hotel Tahara's, P.O. Box 1015, Papeete. A magnificent, upside-down hotel overlooking historic Matavai Bay. Lobby is on the top floor, balconied rooms cling to the cliffside, descending to the black sand beach. Swimming pool, golf, trap shooting, tennis. Tahitian music and dancers.

Tahiti Beachcomber Hotel, P.O. Box 6014, Faaa. Deluxe hotel with 183 air-conditioned rooms plus 17 Tahitian-style bungalows, 4½ miles from Papeete. Fine white beach, swimming pool with bar, tennis courts, all water sports, Tahitian entertainment.

THAILAND

One of Asia's loveliest and most interesting countries, with enchanting

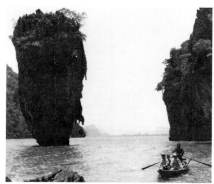

Near Phuket, Thailand.

people, famous for their beauty and courteous dignity. Although Bangkok's noisy traffic and undistinguished buildings make it a rather unattractive city, there are many handsome Buddhist temples worth seeing and, of course, the imposing Palace. Just a two-hour drive away is Pattaya Beach with its sumptuous hotels and a varied selection of nightlife, ranging from Thai boxing exhibits to frenetic discothequing to supper club dining and dancing. Off the coast in the southernmost part of the country is Phuket Island, peaceful and charming, a base for excursions to Phangnga Bay, where *The Man With the Golden Arm* was filmed, and no one there will ever let you forget it.

Royal Cliff Beach Hotel, Pattaya Beach Resort, Cholburi. The only hotel in Pattaya directly on the beach, it's a luxurious self-contained resort with smashingly decorated balconied rooms with views over the Gulf of Siam and the Coral Islands. Two swimming pools, children's pool, bowling alley, parasailing, water scooters, waterskiing, sailing, fishing. Limousine transportation to golf courses.

Phuket Island Resort, 73/1 Rasda Road, Phuket. Hotel rooms and bungalows amid tropical surroundings. Sea View Restaurant built on rocks overlooking the Andaman Sea, beneath the Moon Terrace, built out onto the sea. International and local cuisine featuring famous Phuket lobster. Swimming pool, children's pool, tennis, badminton. Diving club offers snorkeling and scuba diving courses taught by professional European divers.

Appendix: Temperature and Weather Charts

Wherever possible we have given climate information for the specific resorts and locales mentioned in the travel section of this book. When such information was not available we have used the nearest large city as the point of reference.

The information is arranged in this fashion:

Centigrade high (day)	Fahrenheit high (day)
Centigrade low (night)	Fahrenheit low (night)

Average humidity

Number of days in which there is NO RAIN AT ALL. (Certain islands and coastal areas have rain every day but it lasts only a few minutes and otherwise the day is fair and beautiful. The information is given to help guide you in selecting clothing and making general vacation plans.)

UNITED STATES

	Temp: C/F	JAN.	FEB.	MAR.	APR.	MAY	JUN.	JUL.	AUG.	SEP.	OCT.	NOV.	DEC.
	day	-2/29	-1/31	4/40	12/54	19/67	25/77	28/83	26/79	23/74	15/59	7/45	-1/31
BURLINGTON,	night	-12/11	-12/11	-6/22	1/34	7/45	13/56	15/59	14/58	10/50	4/40	-1/31	-9/16
VERMONT	Humidity	72	71	68	67	66	69	69	72	76	74	74	74
	Sun Days	26	24	26	24	25	25	25	25	25	26	26	26
CHARLESTON,		14/58	15/69	19/67	23/74	27/81	30/86	31/88	31/88	28/83	24/76	19/67	15/59
SOUTH CAROLINA		6/43	7/45	10/50	14/58	19/67	23/74	24/76	24/76	22/72	16/61	11/52	7/45
		73	72	71	68	69	71	73	75	76	71	70	73
		25	23	25	24	25	23	21	22	22	26	26	25
CHARLESTON,		10/50	11/52	16/61	21/70	26/79	29/85	32/90	31/88	29/85	22/72	16/61	11/52
WEST VIRGINIA		-3/27	-3/27	2/36	6/43	11/52	16/61	18/65	17/63	14/58	7/45	2/36	-2/29
		24	22	24	23	24	22	23	24	25	26	26	25
PHOENIX,		18/64	21/69	24/75	28/82	33/91	38/100	40/104	38/100	36/96	30/86	24/75	19/66
ARIZONA		4/39	6/42	8/46	12/53	16/60	21/69	25/77	24/75	21/69	13/55	7/44	4/39
		54	51	45	36	29	26	39	44	42	43	51	54
		29	27	29	29	31	30	28	28	28	29	28	29
TUCSON,		18/64	20/68	23/73	28/82	32/89	37/98	38/100	36/96	29/84	29/84	23/73	19/66
ARIZONA		3/37	4/39	7/44	11/51	14/57	19/66	23/73	20/68	14/57	14/57	7/44	4/39
		47	41	33	26	20	21	43	33	34	34	41	44
		29	27	29	29	31	30	26	29	28	29	28	29
LOS ANGELES,		18/64	18/64	19/66	19/66	21/69	22/71	24/75	24/75	24/75	23/73	22/71	19/66
CALIFORNIA		7/44	8/46	9/48	11/51	12/53	14/57	16/60	17/62	16/60	13/55	9/48	8/46
		68	66	70	72	72	75	75	76	75	73	64	64
		25	23	26	27	31	30	31	31	30	30	28	26
PALM SPRINGS,		21/69	23/73	26/78	30/86	34/93	39/102	42/107	41/105	39/102	33/91	26/78	21/69
CALIFORNIA		4/39	7/44	8/46	11/51	14/57	18/64	23/73	22/71	19/66	14/57	9/48	6/42
		43	46	40	34	33	33	29	32	32	33	38	49
		28	26	29	29	31	30	30	30	29	30	23	28
COLORADO SPRINGS,		6/42	8/46	9/48	14/57	20/68	27/80	29/84	28/82	25/77	18/64	11/51	8/46
COLORADO		-9/15	-7/19	-5/23	0/32	6/42	11/51	13/55	13/55	8/46	3/37	-4/24	-7/19
		57	59	53	56	56	49	53	54	48	53	55	58
		30	28	29	26	5	26	26	26	27	2 9	28	30
LAS VEGAS,		16/60	19/66	22/71	27/80	32/89	37/98	39/102	39/102	35/95	29/84	22/71	16/60
NEVADA		-2/28	1/33	4/39	7/44	11/51	16/60	20/68	19/66	14/57	8/46	2/35	-1/30
		46	41	34	29	22	18	22	24	22	29	37	48
		30	29	30	30	31	29	29	30	29	30	29	30
SANTA FE,		4/39	6/42	11/51	15/59	20/68	26/78	27/80	26/78	23/73	17/62	10/50	4/39
NEW MEXICO		-7/19	-5/23	-2/28	2/35	6/42	11/51	14/57	13/55	9/48	3/37	-2/28	-7/19
		58	58	53	46	40	39	50	52	51	49	51	60
		29	27	29	29	29	28	26	25	28	29	29	30
CHEYENNE,		2/35	3/37	7/44	12/53	17/62	23/73	27/80	26/78	22/71	14/57	8/46	4/39
WYOMING		-9/15	-9/15	-6/21	-2/28	3/37	8/46	12/53	11/51	6/42	0/32	-5/23	-8/17
		55	57	58	60	60	56	55	55	53	55	54	56
		29	27	28	26	24	25	27	28	28	29	28	29

BAHAMAS, BERMUDA, & THE CARIBBEAN

	Temp: C/F	JAN.	FEB.	MAR.	APR.	MAY	JUN.	JUL.	AUG.	SEP.	OCT.	NOV.	DEC.
	day	25/77	25/77	26/79	27/81	29/85	31/88	31/88	32/90	31/88	29/85	27/81	26/79
BAHAMAS:	night	18/65	18/65	19/67	21/70	22/72	23/74	24/76	24/76	34/76	23/74	21/70	19/67
NASSAU	Humidity	74	72	73	72	72	75	75	76	79	77	76	75
	Sun Days	25	24	26	24	22	18	17	17	15	17	22	25
		19/67	19/67	19/67	21/70	23/74	26/79	28/83	29/85	28/83	26/79	23/74	21/70
BERMUDA:		16/61	16/61	16/60	17/63	19/67	22/72	24/76	25/77	24/76	22/72	19/67	17/63
ST. GEORGES		72	72	70	73	78	82	78	77	76	75	71	71
		20	21	22	24	25	22	23	23	20	21	22	21
		27/81	27/81	28/83	28/83	29/85	29/85	30/86	30/86	30/86	30/86	29/85	28/83
ANTIGUA:		22/72	22/72	22/72	23/74	24/76	25/77	25/77	25/77	24/76	24/76	24/76	23/74
ST. JOHN'S		76	74	73	73	77	77	77	78	78	80	79	78
		24	25	28	27	25	23	24	23	23	22	22	24
		28/83	28/83	29/85	30/86	31/88	31/88	30/86	31/88	31/88	30/86	29/85	28/83
BARBADOS:		21/70	21/70	21/70	22/72	23/74	23/74	23/74	23/74	23/74	23/74	23/74	22/72
BRIDGETOWN		73	69	67	66	68	71	73	74	75	77	79	75
		18	21	23	24	23	16	13	15	15	16	15	17
		28/83	28/83	29/85	29/85	29/85	29/85	30/86	32/90	32/90	32/90	29/85	29/85
DOMINICAN REPUBLIC:		23/74	24/76	24/76	23/74	23/74	23/74	24/76	26/79	26/79	26/79	24/76	24/76
HIGÜEY		87	83	85	83	84	85	84	85	82	83	80	85
		13	12	23	14	19	19	16	17	12	9	9	22
		29/85	29/85	29/85	29/85	30/86	30/86	30/86	28/88	30/86	30/86	30/86	29/85
GRENADA:		24/76	24/76	24/76	25/77	26/79	25/77	25/77	25/77	24/76	24/76	25/77	24/76
ST. GEORGES		71	70	71	75	74	78	78	74	79	79	77	74
		18	17	23	16	17	7	7	8	8	9	10	13
		28/83	28/83	29/85	29/85	30/86	31/88	31/88	31/88	31/88	31/88	29/85	29/85
GUADELOUPE:		19/67	19/67	19/67	21/70	22/72	23/74	23/74	23/74	22/72	22/72	21/70	20/68
POINTE-À-PITRE		82	81	77	77	81	81	80	83	85	85	85	84
		20	23	25	22	20	18	17	17	16	16	17	19
		31/88	31/88	32/90	32/90	32/90	33/92	34/94	34/94	33/92	32/90	31/88	31/88
HAITI:		20/68	20/68	21/70	22/72	22/72	23/74	23/74	23/74	23/74	22/72	22/72	21/70
PORT-AU-PRINCE		58	58	58	60	65	61	56	11	65	68	66	61
		28	24	24	19	·18	22	24	20	18	19	23	28
		30/86	30/86	31/88	31/88	32/90	31/88	32/90	32/90	32/90	32/90	32/90	29/85
JAMAICA:		21/70	22/72	22/72	23/74	23/24	24/76	23/74	23/74	24/76	23/74	23/74	21/70
MONTEGO BAY		76	73	71	76	76	77	77	80	80	81	79	76
		25	28	25	23	23	18	20	15	20	14	16	25
		30/86	29/85	29/85	30/86	31/88	31/88	31/88	31/88	31/88	31/88	30/86	29/85
JAMAICA:		22/72	22/72	23/74	23/74	24/76	25/77	25/77	25/77	23/74	23/74	22/72	22/72
OCHO RIOS		73	74	74	75	77	76	75	77	78	78	75	74
		30	28	30	27	25	20	26	20	20	22	26	29
		28/83	29/85	29/85	30/86	31/88	30/86	30/86	31/88	31/88	31/88	30/86	29/85
MARTINIQUE:		21/70	21/70	21/70	22/72	23/74	23/74	23/74	23/74	23/74	23/74	22/72	22/72
PORT-DU-FRANCE		84	81	80	80	81	83	84	85	81	86	87	85
		12	14	16	17	13	9	9	9	1	12	10	12

CARIBBEAN

Temp: C/F		JAN.	FEB.	MAR.	APR.	MAY	JUN.	JUL.	AUG.	SEP.	OCT.	NOV.	DEC.
	day	27/81	27/81	27/81	28/83	29/85	29/85	29/85	29/85	30/86	29/85	29/85	27/81
PUERTO RICO:	night	21/70	21/70	21/70	22/72	23/74	24/76	24/76	24/76	24/76	24/76	23/74	22/72
SAN JUAN	Humidity	78	77	75	75	76	77	78	78	78	78	78	79
	Sun Days	11	14	16	16	15	13	12	12	12	13	11	9
		28/83	27/81	29/85	29/85	29/85	30/86	30/86	31/88	31/88	30/86	29/85	27/81
ST. MARTIN/ST. MAARTEN		22/72	22/72	22/72	23/74	23/74	24/76	24/76	24/76	24/76	23/74	22/72	22/72
PHILIPSBURG		71	70	67	69	69	70	69	70	71	72	70	71
		20	16	23	22	21	24	19	16	21	18	20	16
		31/88	31/88	32/90	32/90	32/90	32/92	31/88	31/88	32/90	32/90	32/90	31/88
TRINIDAD:		21/70	20/68	20/68	21/70	22/72	22/72	22/72	22/72	22/72	22/72	22/72	21/70
PORT-OF-SPAIN		79	76	74	72	74	78	80	80	80	81	83	80
		17	19	2	21	18	11	9	8	11	13	12	14
		29/85	29/85	29/85	30/86	31/88	31/88	31/88	32/90	32/90	31/88	30/86	29/85
U.S. VIRGIN ISLANDS:		22/72	22/72	22/72	23/74	23/74	24/76	24/76	24/76	24/76	24/76	23/74	22/72
ST. CROIX		76	75	74	76	78	77	78	79	79	80	80	79
		25	24	27	24	24	23	22	26	21	22	22	23

MEXICO

Temp: C/F		JAN.	FEB.	MAR.	APR.	MAY	JUN.	JUL.	AUG.	SEP.	OCT.	NOV.	DEC.
	day	31/88	31/88	31/88	31/88	32/90	32/90	33/91	33/91	32/90	3/90	32/90	31/88
ACAPULCO	night	22/72	22/72	22/72	23/73	25/77	25/77	25/77	25/77	25/77	25/77	24/75	23/73
	Humidity	75	74	74	75	74	76	76	76	78	78	76	76
	Sun Days	30	29	31	30	29	17	18	18	14	23	28	30
		24/75	25/77	28/82	30/86	31/88	29/84	26/79	26/79	26/79	26/79	25/77	24/75
GUADALAJARA		7/45	8/46	9/48	12/54	14/57	16/61	15/59	15/59	15/59	12/54	9/48	8/46
		52	46	41	37	42	61	71	73	73	66	58	56
		29	27	30	29	26	14	8	11	12	23	28	28
		30/86	29/85	30/86	30/86	32/89	33/91	34/93	34/93	32/90	33/91	32/89	31/87
MANZANILLO		20/68	19/67	19/66	19/67	22/71	24/76	24/76	24/76	24/76	24/76	23/73	21/70
		76	78	76	77	82	86	87	85	85	84	83	78
		30	29	31	30	31	22	21	22	19	26	29	30
		21/70	23/73	26/79	27/81	26/79	25/77	23/73	23/72	22/72	22/72	22/72	21/70
MEXICO CITY		5/41	7/45	9/48	10/50	11/52	12/54	11/52	11/52	11/52	10/50	7/45	6/43
		54	48	44	45	53	64	72	72	72	66	61	58
		29	27	28	22	18	12	8	9	11	22	26	28
		29/84	30/86	30/86	31/88	33/91	34/93	35/95	35/95	34/93	34/93	33/91	30/86
PUERTO VALLARTA		17/63	16/61	17/63	18/64	20/68	23/73	23/73	23/73	23/73	22/72	20/68	18/64
		30	28	30	30	30	18	13	13	12	24	29	30

SOUTH AMERICA

	Temp: C/F	JAN.	FEB.	MAR.	APR.	MAY	JUN.	JUL.	AUG.	SEP.	OCT.	NOV.	DEC.
ARGENTINA:	day	29/85	28/83	26/79	22/72	18/64	14/57	14/57	16/60	18/64	21/69	24/76	28/82
	night	17/63	17/63	16/69	12/53	8/47	5/41	6/42	6/43	8/64	10/50	13/56	16/61
BUENOS AIRES	Humidity	71	73	78	80	82	85	86	82	77	74	70	71
	Sun Days	24	23	24	22	24	23	23	22	22	23	21	23
BRAZIL:		25/77	26/79	24/76	23/73	20/68	19/66	19/66	19/66	19/67	0/68	22/72	24/75
SÃO PAULO		17/63	18/64	17/62	15/59	12/54	12/54	12/53	12/53	13/55	14/57	15/59	17/62
		82	83	81	82	80	79	75	73	77	78	80	80
		19	18	23	26	26	26	28	27	24	24	22	19
BRAZIL:		30/86	30/86	30/86	29/85	28/83	28/82	27/80	27/81	28/82	29/84	29/85	29/82
RECIFE		25/77	25/77	24/76	24/75	23/74	23/73	22/71	22/71	23/73	24/75	24/76	25/71
		73	76	76	78	79	80	78	78	74	71	71	77
		21	17	17	13	19	9	9	12	19	23	23	17
BRAZIL:		29/84	29/85	28/83	27/80	25/77	24/76	24/75	24/76	24/75	25/77	26/79	28/82
RIO DE JANEIRO		33/73	33/73	22/72	21/69	19/66	18/64	17/63	18/64	18/65	19/66	20/68	22/71
		76	78	81	80	79	78	77	75	78	78	77	77
		18	18	19	20	21	23	24	24	19	17	17	17
ECUADOR:		30/86	30/86	31/88	30/86	30/83	28/81	27/81	27/81	27/81	27/81	27/81	28/83
GALAPAGOS ISLANDS		22/72	24/76	24/76	24/76	23/74	22/72	21/70	19/67	19/67	19/67	20/68	21/70
		23	20	25	24	27	26	22	23	23	29	26	25

EUROPE

	Temp:C/F	JAN.	FEB.	MAR.	APR.	MAY	JUN.	JUL.	AUG.	SEP.	OCT.	NOV.	DEC.
AUSTRIA:	day	1/34	4/39	11/52	16/61	20/68	24/75	25/77	24/75	21/70	15/59	8/46	2/36
	night	-7/19	-5/23	0/32	4/39	8/46	11/52	13/55	12/54	10/50	5/41	0/32	-4/25
INNSBRUCK	Humidity	77	72	65	63	62	66	69	70	72	73	77	79
	Sun Days	8	16	20	16	16	11	12	14	16	19	18	18
AUSTRIA:		1/34	1/34	3/37	15/59	18/64	17/63	23/73	23/73	17/63	14/57	5/41	1/34
KITZBÜHEL (TIROL)		-9/16	-6/21	-6/21	4/39	10/50	12/54	14/57	14/57	7/45	10/50	-1/30	-4/25
		84	84	77	70	74	78	69	74	79	76	85	89
		30	15	19	24	18	10	23	16	19	29	20	21
FRANCE:		6/43	6/43	9/48	12/54	15/59	18/64	20/68	20/68	18/64	14/57	10/50	7/45
BEAULIEU-SUR-MER		2/26	2/36	3/37	6/43	9/48	12/54	14/57	14/57	13/55	10/50	6/43	3/37
		87	85	82	79	80	82	83	84	83	83	85	87
		13	15	18	16	18	19	19	18	16	17	14	13
FRANCE:		11/52	12/54	15/59	16/61	18/64	22/72	23/73	24/75	22/72	17/66	15/59	12/54
BIARRITZ		4/39	4/39	6/43	8/46	11/52	14/57	16/61	16/61	15/59	11/52	7/45	5/41
		78	71	71	75	78	79	81	80	81	80	79	79
		15	15	18	15	14	16	18	18	16	16	14	14
FRANCE:		13/55	13/55	15/59	17/63	20/68	24/75	27/81	27/81	25/77	21/70	17/63	13/55
NICE		4/39	9/41	7/45	9/48	13/55	16/61	18/64	18/64	16/61	12/54	8/46	5/41
		68	68	73	75	75	75	72	74	73	72	70	69
		22	22	23	21	23	25	29	27	23	22	21	22

EUROPE

	Temp: C/F	JAN.	FEB.	MAR.	APR.	MAY	JUN.	JUL.	AUG.	SEP.	OCT.	NOV.	DEC.
	day	11/52	12/54	13/55	18/64	23/73	27/81	30/86	30/86	26/79	22/72	16/61	13/55
GREECE:	night	6/43	6/43	7/45	10/50	14/57	18/64	21/70	21/70	18/64	15/59	11/52	8/46
ATHENS	Humidity	77	73	72	70	68	62	58	58	63	72	76	77
	Sun Days	18	21	23	24	26	28	30	30	28	25	22	20
		11/52	12/54	15/59	19/66	23/73	26/79	29/84	29/84	6/79	21/70	16/61	12/54
ITALY:		2/36	3/37	5/41	8/46	12/54	15/59	17/63	17/63	15/59	11/52	7/45	4/39
MONTECATINI													
		22	20	23	22	24	24	29	27	24	23	19	20
		16/61	16/61	17/63	20/68	24/75	27/81	30/86	30/86	28/82	25/77	21/70	18/64
ITALY:		8/46	8/46	9/48	11/52	14/57	18/64	21/70	21/70	19/66	16/61	12/54	10/50
PALERMO		72	68	66	65	65	61	58	58	60	67	69	70
		19	21	23	24	28	28	31	29	26	23	22	21
		6/43	8/46	12/54	17/63	25/77	27/81	27/81	24/75	19/66	12/54	12/54	8/46
ITALY:		1/34	2/36	5/41	10/50	17/63	19/66	18/64	16/61	11/52	7/45	7/45	3/37
VENICE		81	78	77	77	74	73	74	76	78	82	82	84
		25	23	24	21	23	23	24	26	24	22	21	23
		12/54	13/55	14/57	16/61	19/66	23/73	26/79	26/79	24/75	20/68	16/61	14/57
MONACO:		8/46	8/46	10/50	12/52	15/59	19/66	22/72	22/72	20/68	16/61	12/54	10/50
MONTE CARLO		67	70	74	75	77	77	75	74	74	72	72	72
		26	24	23	25	26	26	30	29	26	24	23	25
		14/57	15/59	17/63	20/68	21/70	25/77	27/81	28/82	26/79	22/72	17/63	15/59
PORTUGAL:		8/46	8/47	10/50	12/54	13/55	15/59	17/63	17/63	17/63	14/57	11/52	9/48
LISBON		78	72	71	63	63	60	55	57	62	67	75	78
		16	17	17	20	21	25	29	29	24	22	17	16
		18/64	18/64	19/66	20/68	22/72	22/72	24/75	25/77	25/77	24/75	2/72	19/66
PORTUGAL:		14/57	14/57	14/57	15/59	15/59	16/61	18/64	19/66	18/64	18/64	15/59	14/57
MADEIRA		80	70	71	69	67	74	78	76	71	69	71	69
		12	23	20	26	30	30	31	30	30	26	20	21
		-3/27	-4/25	0/32	6/43	14/57	19/66	22/72	20/68	15/59	8/46	3/37	-1/30
FINLAND:		-9/16	-9/16	-7/19	-1/30	4/39	9/48	13/55	12/54	8/46	3/37	-1/30	-5/23
HELSINKI		88	86	78	74	64	66	70	75	81	85	83	90
		11	11	17	18	19	17	17	16	15	13	11	11
		1/34	1/34	3/37	8/46	14/57	18/64	21/70	20/68	11/52	6/43	6/43	3/37
SWEDEN:		-3/27	-4/25	-2/28	1/34	5/41	10/50	14/57	13/55	6/43	3/37	3/37	0/32
VISBY		85	83	81	75	71	73	75	78	82	86	86	86
		13	14	19	20	22	21	20	19	16	15	14	13
		12/54	13/55	14/57	17/63	21/70	25/77	29/84	28/82	25/77	21/70	17/63	14/57
YUGOSLAVIA:		6/43	6/43	8/46	11/52	14/57	18/64	21/70	21/70	18/64	14/57	10/50	8/46
DUBROVNIK		61	64	64	67	69	65	64	59	63	64	66	66
		18	16	20	20	21	24	27	28	23	20	14	16
		-2/29	1/34	3/38	7/45	10/50	15/59	17/63	16/61	10/50	10/50	3/88	-1/31
SWITZERLAND:		-12/11	-11/13	-8/18	-4/25	0/32	4/40	5/41	5/41	-1/31	-1/31	-6/22	-10/14
ST. MORITZ		69	67	69	68	70	70	70	72	75	75	74	73
		21	22	22	23	20	17	24	20	24	25	19	25

AFRICA

	Temp: C/F	JAN.	FEB.	MAR.	APR.	MAY	JUN.	JUL.	AUG.	SEP.	OCT.	NOV.	DEC.
	day	23/74	26/78	31/87	36/96	39/103	42/107	41/106	41/109	39/103	37/98	31/87	25/77
EGYPT:	night	10/50	11/52	14/58	19/66	23/74	26/78	26/79	26/79	24/75	22/71	17/62	12/53
ASWAN-LUXOR	Humidity	41	34	27	22	22	21	24	26	28	31	36	41
	Sun Days	31	29	31	30	30	30	31	31	30	31	30	31
		31/88	32/90	32/90	32/90	31/88	29/84	28/82	28/82	8/82	29/84	31/88	31/88
IVORY COAST:		23/73	24/75	24/75	24/75	24/75	23/73	23/73	22/72	23/73	23/73	23/73	23/73
ABIDJAN		85	83	83	83	85	89	86	87	88	87	84	84
		28	25	25	21	15	12	23	24	22	18	17	25
		18/65	20/68	23/74	26/79	29/84	13/92	38/101	38/101	33/92	28/83	23/73	19/66
MOROCCO:		4/40	6/43	19/48	11/52	14/57	17/62	19/67	20/68	17/63	14/57	9/49	6/42
MARRAKECH		77	73	70	65	60	58	53	53	57	66	65	71
		4	24	25	24	29	29	30	30	27	27	27	24
		26/79	27/81	27/81	27/81	29/84	31/88	31/88	31/88	32/90	32/90	30/86	27/81
SENEGAL:		18/64	17/63	18/64	18/64	20/68	23/73	24/75	24/75	24/75	24/75	23/73	19/66
DAV-AR		58	63	69	71	73	74	75	81	80	76	65	58
		31	29	31	30	31	29	24	18	19	28	29	31
		26/79	26/79	25/77	22/72	19/67	18/65	17/62	18/65	18/65	21/70	23/74	24/76
SOUTH AFRICA:		16/60	16/60	14/57	12/54	9/49	8/47	7/45	8/47	9/49	11/51	13/55	14/57
CAPE TOWN		63	66	71	75	78	78	79	78	75	69	65	63

MIDDLE EAST

	Temp: C/F	JAN.	FEB.	MAR.	APR.	MAY	JUN.	JUL.	AUG.	SEP.	OCT.	NOV.	DEC.
	day	21/70	23/74	26/79	31/88	35/95	39/103	40/104	40/104	37/99	33/92	28/83	23/74
ISRAEL:	night	9/49	11/52	13/56	17/63	21/70	24/74	25/77	26/79	23/74	21/70	16/61	12/54
EILAT	Humidity	50	46	38	33	30	28	30	33	42	40	45	48
	Sun Days	31	29	31	29	31	30	31	31	30	31	29	30

FAR EAST

	Temp: C/F	JAN.	FEB.	MAR.	APR.	MAY	JUN.	JUL.	AUG.	SEP.	OCT.	NOV.	DEC.
	day	30/86	31/87	32/89	33/91	33/91	32/89	31/88	31/88	31/88	31/88	31/87	31/88
PHILIPPINES:	night	23/74	23/74	23/74	24/75	24/75	24/75	24/75	24/75	24/75	23/74	23/74	24/75
CEBU CITY	Humidity	76	76	73	70	73	77	79	79	79	81	79	77
	Sun Days	23	23	27	27	24	21	22	23	21	21	22	21
		30/86	31/88	33/91	34/93	34/93	33/91	31/88	31/88	31/88	31/88	31/88	30/86
PHILIPPINES:		21/70	21/70	22/72	23/74	24/75	24/75	24/75	24/75	24/75	23/74	22/72	1/70
MANILA		76	74	70	70	75	80	83	83	83	82	80	79
		25	26	27	26	19	13	7	8	8	12	16	20
		30/86	31/88	31/88	31/88	31/88	29/84	29/84	29/84	29/84	29/84	29/84	29/84
SRI LANKA:		22/72	22/72	23/73	24/75	26/79	25/77	25/77	25/77	25/77	24/75	23/73	22/72
COLOMBO		70	69	69	72	77	79	78	77	76	77	76	72
		24	23	23	16	12	12	19	20	17	12	14	21
		32/89	32/91	34/93	35/95	34/93	33/91	32/89	32/89	32/89	31/88	31/88	31/88
THAILAND:		20/68	22/72	24/75	25/77	25/77	24/75	24/75	24/75	24/75	24/75	22/72	20/68
BANGKOK		72	74	74	74	78	79	79	79	82	82	79	74
		30	28	28	27	22	20	18	18	15	16	25	30

INDIA

	Temp: C/F	JAN.	FEB.	MAR.	APR.	MAY	JUN.	JUL.	AUG.	SEP.	OCT.	NOV.	DEC.
GOA	day	29/84	29/84	31/88	32/90	32/90	31/88	29/84	28/83	28/83	29/84	30/86	29/84
	night	21/70	22/72	24/75	26/79	27/81	25/77	24/75	25/75	24/75	24/75	23/73	21/70
	Humidity	64	69	71	73	74	85	87	88	86	80	67	61
	Sun Days	31	29	31	29	28	9	6	8	15	5	20	31
JAIPUR		23/73	26/79	32/90	37/99	41/106	39/102	34/93	32/90	34/93	34/93	29/84	24/75
		8/46	11/52	16/61	21/70	26/79	27/81	26/79	24/75	23/73	18/64	12/54	9/48
		42	36	25	20	25	41	65	70	59	35	35	42
		30	28	30	29	29	26	21	21	25	30	30	30
MADRAS		29/84	31/88	33/91	35/95	38/100	38/100	36/97	35/95	34/93	32/90	29/84	29/84
		19/66	20/68	22/72	26/79	28/82	27/81	26/79	26/79	25/77	24/75	22/72	21/70
		77	75	74	73	65	60	64	69	73	79	81	80
		29	28	31	29	30	27	23	23	23	20	19	26
UDAIPUR		23/74	28/83	34/94	38/101	36/97	30/86	30/86	32/90	33/92	29/85	29/85	27/81
		6/43	10/50	16/61	22/72	25/77	24/76	23/74	22/72	16/61	9/49	9/49	8/47
		48	46	34	23	48	76	85	72	45	42	42	45
		31	29	31	30	26	23	25	23	31	30	30	31
BOMBAY		28/82	28/82	30/86	32/90	33/91	32/90	29/84	29/84	29/84	32/90	32/90	31/88
		19/66	19/66	22/72	4/74	27/81	26/79	25/77	24/75	24/75	24/75	23/73	21/70
		66	67	69	71	71	78	83	82	82	76	69	66
		31	29	31	30	30	16	10	11	17	28	29	31

ASIA & THE PACIFIC

	Temp: C/F												
AUSTRALIA:	day	32/90	32/90	31/88	29/85	27/81	26/79	26/79	27/81	28/83	30/86	31/88	32/90
CAIRNS	night	23/74	23/74	23/74	21/70	19/67	18/65	16/61	17/63	18/65	20/68	21/70	23/74
	Humidity	72	72	74	73	73	72	69	67	65	65	65	18
	Sun Days	15	13	12	15	19	20	23	23	23	24	20	19
HAWAII:		24/76	24/76	25/77	26/79	27/81	27/81	28/83	28/83	28/83	28/83	27/81	26/79
HONOLULU, OAHU		21/70	19/67	19/67	20/68	21/70	22/72	23/74	23/74	23/74	22/72	21/70	21/70
		71	71	69	67	67	66	67	68	68	70	71	72
		29	27	30	30	29	30	30	31	30	29	24	23
HONG KONG		18/65	17/62	19/66	24/75	28/82	29/84	31/88	31/88	29/84	27/80	23/74	20/68
		13/56	13/56	16/60	19/66	23/74	26/78	26/78	26/78	25/77	23/74	18/65	15/59
		72	78	79	82	83	82	82	82	78	69	67	69
		27	24	24	22	18	12	14	16	18	25	29	28
MACAU		20/68	20/68	21/70	23/74	28/82	29/84	31/88	31/88	30/86	28/82	25/77	20/68
		13/56	15/59	16/60	20/68	23/74	25/77	26/78	26/78	24/75	23/74	20/68	14/57
		73	87	82	91	83	88	85	80	82	79	79	80
		30	22	27	17	20	11	10	3	18	22	25	27

185

PHOTO ACKNOWLEDGEMENTS

Willie Allegne Associates; Air France; American Museum of Natural History; Australian Tourist Commission; Austrian National Tourist Office; Bermuda News Bureau; The Bettman Archive; Bonaire Tourist Information Office; British Tourist Authority; Casa de Campo Hotel, Villas and Country Club; French West Indies Tourist Board; German Information Center; Greek National Tourist Office; Hawaii Visitors Bureau; Italian Government Travel Office; KLM; Little Dix Bay, British Virgin Islands; Portugese National Tourist Office; South African Tourist Corporation; Swiss National Tourist Office; Tunisian National Tourist Office; Turkish Tourism and Information Office; U.S. Virgin Islands Tourist Board; Ray Cranborne, p. 176; Michele Renandean, p. 172.

Eleanor Bach, an astrologer active in The Astrologer's Guild and The National Council for Geo-Cosmic Research, gave much valuable guidance in the writing of Chapter 9. She is the author of *Ceres, Pallas, Juno, and Vesta,* a text for astrologers which gives the Zodiacal position of four tiny planets known as the asteroids.